Muted Consent

Science and Society:
A Purdue University Series in Science,
Technology, and Human Values

Leon E. Trachtman, General Editor

Volume 1

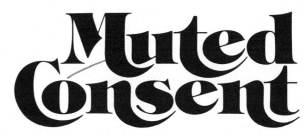

Muted Consent

A Casebook in Modern Medical Ethics

by Jan Wojcik

Purdue University
West Lafayette, Indiana
1978

Any opinions, findings, conclusions, or recommendations expressed herein are those of the author and do not necessarily reflect the views of the National Endowment for the Humanities.

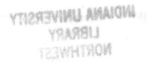

Library of Congress Card Catalog Number 77-89472

Printed in the United States of America

For Lorraine, who knows ethics

Contents

Acknowledgments

Leon Trachtman, associate dean of the School of Humanities, Social Science, and Education at Purdue University, wrote the grant proposal for a series of seminars and studies bearing on the impact of modern technology on human values. He administered the grant and gave frequent wise counsel to the seminar in the series out of which this book grew. Daniel Hartl, a geneticist and an associate professor of biology at Purdue was the member of the team teaching the seminar who made intelligible the scientific matters discussed in class and in this book. The practical experience of Alan A. Alexander, M.D., and attorney John McBride, both of whom also helped us teach, gave the discussion life. Jeffrey Smalldon gathered data, ran down leads, conferred with knowledgeable sources, and typed the manuscript over and over. The packets of readings on medical ethics put out by the Institute of Society, Ethics, and the Life Sciences, Hastings-on-Hudson, New York, made readily available much material from which this review drew. Helen Wojcik rearranged the prose until it made some sense.

This volume was developed and produced with the assistance of an educational grant from the National Endowment for the Humanities, #EH-10433-74-443.

Introduction

Consentless Medicine

The Issues

The consent of the patient always has been the bedrock of
ethical medicine. A physician informs a patient what promise
and risk a cure involves; a patient freely decides whether the
promise is worth the risk. Informed consent is still common.
It is silently assumed in routine visits to a doctor's office. It
is explicit and often put into writing before a serious operation
or before an untried drug is prescribed. Outright violations of
the canon of fidelity binding patient and physician have been infrequent and, when made public, are roundly condemned:
witness the outrage at the worst horrors of Nazi medicine and
at the experiments at Willowbrook Hospital in New York where
mentally retarded children were deliberately infected with hepatitis. (There is a discussion of these cases in Chapter One.)

But in recent years, as medicine has learned more and more
about how bodies grow and work and heal, the number of its
potential experimental subjects or patients has grown larger
than the relatively small number of people informed enough to
consent freely or to be consented for by well-meaning guardians.
Modern medical techniques literally manufacture new kinds of
patients mute for consent: consider a living fetus on the
operating table after an abortion, or vulnerable to tests and
probes while in the womb; a "living" cadaver whose brain is
dead but whose heart and lungs a respirator keeps pumping; a
terribly deformed infant who will die soon after birth unless it
receives massive doses of antibiotics. Even alert adults cannot consent to everything modern medicine has to offer. Two
men applying for the use of a single hemodialysis machine could
not be expected to consent to their selection or rejection for

1

treatment. Their consent, although still conceivable, would be muted, "muffled" by the circumstance. Similarly a prisoner perhaps cannot be expected to consent freely to a dangerous medical experiment which promises to advance medical knowledge only at enormous risk to the subject when the prisoner hopes volunteering will win him favor with the parole board. In fact, few educated patients who are not themselves highly trained physicians can understand all the implications and risks of many of the extraordinarily complex procedures modern medicine has developed for curing diseases and altering consciousness and human biology.

In this unsettling atmosphere, the discussion often becomes turbid. The now widely available techniques of newly legalized abortion stir up passionate debates in the courts about the point at which the mother's freedom over her own biology ends and the fetus's right to life begins. The new technology of organ transplants raises tricky legal questions about whether it is perfected enough to be considered "ordinary" and how to determine the precise moment when a potential organ donor dies so that fresh organs can be removed from a bona fide cadaver dead by natural means. A woman lying in a coma for several months hooked up to a respirator becomes a national celebrity when her parents ask her doctors to let her die a natural death, when the doctors refuse, and when a court upholds their decision against the parents' wishes. Many people are outraged when a doctor who performs a legal abortion is tried and convicted of manslaughter for killing the viable fetus he aborted. The initial successes scientists have had in genetic engineering, now mostly on the level of using amniocentesis to determine whether or not a fetus is "defective," and in cloning (reproducing a biological replica of an organism from a single parent cell) raises nervous questions as to whether such research should continue at all. Will the world be able to handle machine-made human beings?

The Goal of This Book

This book was conceived in order to clarify the issues raised by medicine's growing capabilities to touch and change mankind. The remainder of the Introduction examines the underlying structure of the medical ethics debate. Each chapter begins with three fictional cases illustrating the sorts of dilemmas that can arise in one of seven areas of modern medicine: experimentation with human subjects; genetic counseling and screening; abortion; behavior modification with drugs, surgery, and psychology; the treatment of the dying and dead; the allocation of scarce medical resources; and genetic engineering. The major part of each chapter reviews a broad range of the best thinking about the ethics of each area of medicine, in order to supply the reader with ideas with which to puzzle out an opinion about the ethics involved in each case; the book draws no conclusions of its own. It is hoped that the book will be used as a primer in the language of medical ethics, a language we all must understand if we are to make sense out of the private and public dilemmas modern medical progress will almost certainly bring our way.

The Structure of the Medical Ethics Debate

People worrying about consentless medicine tend to follow the bent of one of two biblically rooted paradigms. One line of thinking emerges from the belief that humans have only limited control over their own fate. Destiny or Providence brings them into being at a certain time; they live according to plans or designs not wholly within their control; their limited nature is nowhere more obvious than when at a certain time and place they cease to be. They were, after all, only made "in the image of God," not as God. Relevant to consentless medicine, this belief would sometimes predispose a person to let nature take its course when a particular patient is mute for consent. The fetus would be allowed to grow, the comatose patient allowed to die. It would incline a physician to recognize sickness or abnormality as a limitation analogous to his or her own mortality. An insane or retarded or imprisoned person would be considered to be as fully human as the physician or medical experimenter.

Another line of thinking follows from believing that humans become human insofar as they master their own fate and rationally civilize the jungle and sea and their own violent or egotistical impulses. Humans were driven from Eden to work

things out for themselves, with sickness and death as their
natural enemies. Relevant to consentless medicine, this belief
would predispose a person to modify rationally unfortunate
circumstances. A woman's rational decision not to have a child
would be allowed to counter the natural forces threatening to
deliver her of one; artificial respiration can keep a patient
"alive" until fresh organs are needed for a transplant; as intervention via medication was once appropriate to allow diabetics
to live normal lives, intervention via genetic engineering is
now appropriate to lessen the number of future diabetics. This
belief would incline a researcher to regard an insane or retarded
or imprisoned person if not necessarily less human than he
or she, at least more worthy the more useful they could be in
helping research to advance human knowledge. Consentful
medicine is not a necessary ideal; more important a patient
than a man is mankind.[1]

It is rare that anyone draws such fundamental structures to
the surface of their thinking. Paul Ramsey and Joseph Fletcher,
cited frequently in these pages, often come close, though even
their arguments are too complex to be so simply reducible.[2]
It is more important to see how one assumption would work to
give ethical direction in a complex practical situation.

Despite their limitations, however, the two paradigms open
some windows where there would otherwise be walls. They show
us, for example, that we are often like amphibians, dividing
loyalties between these two different definitions of ourselves.
A woman wonders whether she can bear the burden in her busy
life of raising a retarded child, or the burden on her moral
conscience if she doesn't. A legislator might wonder whether
the widespread practice of abortion promises at last a practical, safe solution to the age-old human problem of unwanted
children, or signifies a decreasingly humane sensibility. A
dying patient's final serenity falters when he is tempted by the
promise which heroic medicine gives him to live a little bit
longer a quasi-mechanical existence. A man with a kidney
disease tries to decide whether to discontinue the painful dialysis treatment he needs to live, but which is draining his
family's financial reserves. In such cases, freedom to make a
decision can be terrible. There is no automatic solution. If

one seeks advice widely enough it will be contradictory. Finally, one must make a fundamental decision on what human life or one's own life means, abandoned by the comforting or sentimental answers that serve well enough in times of tranquility.

The two positions highlight the real issues in medical ethics when the patient is altogether mute for consent. Those deciding for the patient fall back on one assumption or the other: deciding to let the biological fate of the fetus or the dying old man run its course, or deciding to thwart fate with an abortion or a respirator for the good of the patient or the family or society or science. We can see why such debates are often endless. People can change sides on an issue, but there is little or no real compromise available between exclusive positions. Arbitration does not really settle such disputes, nor does majority opinion, nor judicial fiat, nor even legal enforcement. Those opposed to abortion continue to fight the recent Supreme Court ruling, just as women continued to seek and to obtain illegal abortions before the ruling. Certain religious sects still refuse blood transfusions for their unconscious ailing members; their doctors still go to court for injunctions to force their acceptance.

There is a special urgency to the clash of the two assumptions where the new medicine merges with the new biology to move it beyond curing to making human beings. As scientists develop techniques for cloning (twinning) human beings, or engineering their biology, we seem as a species to stand on the verge of being able to make human life fit one or the other of these concepts, irrevocably. Because the two positions are really exclusive, it would have to be one or the other; man is going to decide to remain as he has been or become something different (but whether higher or lower is not clear). And what is even more unsettling to those who cherish the first paradigm or assumption is that perhaps there is nothing human beings can do about arresting the human takeover of human destiny; we might already be swept up in the momentum which our curiosity has created, heading towards increasingly "efficient" societies or their transformation before we can decide what we really want. George Steiner writes: "It is as if the biochemical and biogenetic facts and potentialities we are beginning to elucidate were waiting in ambush for man. It may prove to be that the

dilemmas and possibilities of action they will pose are outside
morality and beyond the ordinary grasp of the human intellect. "[3]

But perhaps here as in other areas even a practical compromise is possible. If enough disparate voices join the discussion about what humans should let medicine do to themselves,
their debate would be so complex, their enthusiasm and caution so convoluted, that the decisions arrived at would approximate fate itself: the difference between what humans propose
to do and what after interminable decisions and revisions,
fidgeting and arguing and remeasuring and making qualifications
and compromises, and hunkering down for another look, they
finally wind up being able to do.

Chapter 1

Experimentation on Human Subjects

The Cases

1   A team of scientists is studying the human body's natural tendency to reject foreign tissue. Certain lymphoid tissues in the human body can recognize foreign matter by its antigens and can produce antibodies to stave off the invasion. Other parts of the defense system destroy the invader and record the type of attack and the proper response in order to make future reactions even more immediate and massive. Medical immunization against disease manipulates the system by stimulating it to produce its own antibodies against artificially introduced doses of the disease small enough to be handled easily. But the system frustrates other medical procedures; it attacks organ or tissue transplants as intruders as well.

The scientists have developed a new, sophisticated drug to blunt the body's response. They test it on rats successfully, then devise an experiment using two hundred human subjects. The subjects are to be paired. A tiny skin graft from one will be transplanted to the other. Half the number of those receiving the transplant will be treated with the drug, and the other half, serving as a control group, will not. As a further control of their experiment, fifty pairs or half the number of subjects will be identical twins, each of whose immunization systems recognizes transplanted tissue from the other twin to be identical with its own and usually ignores it. In order to be able to find that many twins who are still living close to each other, the scientists decide to solicit child volunteers for their experiments. They contact parents through the local school system and soon find enough willing to sign consent forms for their children. When the twins are in the middle to late teens, they are also asked to consent to the experiment.

The results of the experiment prove the new drug to work effectively and selectively to blunt the rejection of transplanted tissue. A slightly higher percentage of the treated twins--90 percent versus 86 percent--accept the skin grafts; a much higher percentage of the non-twin treated subjects--80 percent versus 10 percent--accept them.

2   Scientists have discovered that the bodies of rats reject living cancer cells inserted surgically under their skins. Studying the process holds promise of learning how certain natural bodily mechanisms might be used in the fight against cancer. After doing extensive work with animals, several researchers ask permission of the prison authorities in their state to solicit prisoner-volunteers to determine whether the human body might react in similar ways. The researchers are particularly interested in prisoners with long sentences who might be available for long-term observation. No promise is made to the volunteers that they will receive special pay or special consideration from their parole boards. They will, however, be taken from the prison for several periods of several weeks duration to be observed under clinical conditions in a local hospital. A sufficient number of prisoners volunteer. In each case their bodies reject the cancer cells.

3   Scientists are experimenting with a new drug that might offer immunization against rubella (German Measles). They are particularly interested in the problem of pregnant women who have not been previously immunized. The usual vaccine which is quite safe for children and adults has been proved capable of crossing the placenta of a pregnant woman and adversely affecting the fetus. Yet women who are not immunized and who do contact rubella during pregnancy run the risk of bearing deformed children. After discovering that the new vaccine does not cross the placenta of pregnant primates, the researchers ask for permission to try the drug on women who have decided to seek legal abortions for their unwanted fetuses. Sufficient numbers of women volunteer. They are vaccinated. Postmorten analyses of their aborted fetuses show that the drug does cross the placenta of human mothers. It is decided not to recommend its use as an emergency vaccination for unvaccinated mothers.

The Issues

The motives behind medical research have usually been the same. Human beings have always gotten sick; even a perfectly healthy old man eventually must die of something. And so medicine men have continuously wanted to know more about why and the way in which their patients suffer and die. They sympathize with them; they enjoy successful curing and getting paid well for it; they become intrigued by the intricacies of human pathology and mastering the maze of its cure.

Their procedures have likewise been the same. Concocting new theories and medicines from the old, researchers try them out first on less worthy forms of life--presently animals--but at times on slaves or prisoners. Then, inevitably, they try them out for the first time on a "real" human subject, usually someone in great distress whose case is otherwise utterly hopeless. A risk finally must be taken and taken again and again until a procedure becomes commonplace and proven, temporarily at least, to be the best.

The crux of the ethics of medical experimentation on human subjects is how to go about taking risks, which usually boils down to the question of who shall take risks. Should a new procedure or drug be tried out only on patients whose case is otherwise hopeless, or routinely on healthy volunteers whose greater numbers and more regulated treatment could move medical research ahead much faster? With large numbers of subjects there is always the danger that medical research could trample on the dignity of the human subjects at hand in the march towards the health of humanity. Without them research might become too tentative and timid to do anyone much good.

That modern medical research has done much good with its vast use of human subjects is hardly disputable; as the result of experiments involving thousands of subjects, polio, measles, and failing hearts and kidneys no longer can cripple so many. But with the progress has come abuse and, as it has become recognized, growing concern. At the Nuremberg trials after World War II, it was revealed that Nazi doctors had experimented with political prisoners and prisoners of war on how long a man could live in icy water and whether a new drug could stem the bleeding of a patient deliberately mutilated for the experiment. A multitude of prisoners were killed while researchers tried out new techniques of "ktenology, " the term Leo Alexander, a doctor working with the prosecution, gave to the "science of killing. " 1

The enormous increase in experimentation on human subjects since the war has occasionally brought abuses closer to home. In 1963 at the Jewish Chronic Disease Hospital, Brooklyn, N.Y., researchers injected liver cancer cells into the bodies of terminal patients without informing them, for fear of possible "bizarre, defensive reactions" from the patients.2   In 1967 at the Willowbrook State Hospital in Staten Island, N.Y., five hundred mentally retarded children were injected with a live hepatitis virus as part of a research program. In 1972 it became known that four hundred black men in Alabama with syphilis had been studied to map the history of the untreated disease under the false pretense of treatment.3   The Supreme Court's ruling on January 22, 1973, permitting non-therapeutic abortion, coupled with horror stories of brutal experiments on doomed or dying fetuses has raised fears that an epidemic of unethical experiments on human subjects might be brewing.4

Researchers themselves have come to fear the public's overreaction to abuse as much as the public fears abuse itself. In summarizing the talk that had gone on for two days at a Forum of the National Academy of Sciences on Experimentation with Human Subjects, where these cases and the problem of fetal research had been discussed, Howard Hyatt pointed out the discussion had divided the participants into two groups:

The medical researchers,

> who feel that the excesses, while they exist, are in general minimal as compared with the dividends that have been brought to all of us.... They also feel that if the ground rules are changed appreciably, research itself may be threatened. They feel, finally, that the other players on the stage, potential or real, lawyers, chemists, social workers, consumers, have no greater expertise, and often lesser expertise, than physicians or the investigators; and therefore, why change?

and the nonphysicians,

> who are, in general, cognizant of the contributions of medical research, but who are concerned about the abrogation of individual rights.

Hyatt concludes that

> this gulf is not going to be bridged unless we find mechanisms
> for establishing a continuing dialogue between all the people who
> are concerned, a dialogue that introduces each of the people
> involved to the problems, the aspirations, and the concerns of
> the others.[5]

This book begins with a dialogue about experimentation on
human subjects because its language about patient consent, the
balancing of individual and social needs, and the nature of
human and fetal life occurs over and over again in all other
topics of biomedical ethics. In a sense all of these ethical
topics are about experimentation with humans: how medicine
can change the way humans go about living and dying, and even
whether medicine should tinker with the human nature itself.

Therapeutic Research

Therapeutic research on consenting adults concerns
ethicians the least, which is not to say not at all. According
to AMA guidelines, therapeutic experimentation is "clinical
investigation primarily for treatment." A typical example
would be a forty-year-old women who has suffered since child-
hood from bronchial asthma and who has experienced uncomfortable side effects from most of the drugs and treatments
allergists usually prescribe to alleviate its symptoms. Her
physician, a part-time researcher well versed in the current
literature of his field, knows of a new drug that has been
shown to be helpful in cases similar to hers. After carefully
explaining the purpose, promises, and risks of the drug, and
stressing the point that its administration is not yet an accepted
practice, the physician obtains her consent to administer
the drug and to monitor her reactions clinically. She under-
takes the treatment; her symptoms are relieved with no discern-
ible unpleasant side effects; the physician includes her case
in a published review of his experiments with the drug; more
evidence is gathered for the drug's usefulness. In this
hypothetical case, the doctor experiments while treating a
patient. They have a mutual interest in the experiment. The
subject becomes a willing and knowing accomplice to her own
cure, aware of the risk and promise of a new procedure at

the same time. Paul Ramsey would say they have a "covenant relationship" as "joint adventurers."

To be ethical, however, even this case needs a sound scientific setting. David D. Rutstein describes its usual steps: Prior to administering the drug to a human being, the physician needs to research the pertinent literature about the known toxic and therapeutic effects of the substances used in the drug. Experiments should be done with animals whose biological systems would most closely resemble those of a human being in reacting to the drug. If the research and testing suggested that the drug showed great promise and minimal risk, the physician-experimenter would then submit a protocol for an experiment--a research design--for scrutiny by a review board. The board might consist of an ethician, a biostatistician, and several experts in the experimenter's field. After approving the experiment, the board would monitor the entire experiment. The procedure, Rutstein acknowledges, is well accepted among other writers, and indeed is in use in most research hospitals and clinics. He would secure it further with a "second line of defense" that "can be provided by editors and editorial boards of journals that publish scientific reports of human experiments. If higher scientific standards of publication were established and adhered to, it would soon become clear to investigators that improperly designed studies would not be published. Automatically, many human subjects would be protected against participation in unsound and unethical medical research."[6]

Guido Galabresi would further shore up the ethics of medical experimentation by introducing "market control" into the experimental process:

> The basic device would be a compensation fund for subjects injured in unsuccessful experiments. A separate fund would exist at each medical center where experiments on humans were being undertaken. Moneys for the fund could come from two sources--income from successful results of previous experiments, such as new marketable drugs, and grants from government or foundations based on the expectations that the researches undertaken would be more than worth the money used to compensate the subjects who were injured. The effect of such a fund--apart from compensating the victims--would be

to stimulate greater analysis with each medical center of the possible benefits and risks a given experiment entails.[7]

Rutstein and Galabresi's procedures might seem a bit out of place in our hypothetical case of therapeutic experimentation. In our case it would seem that the venerable and valuable concern of the doctor for his or her patient would provide all the ethical safeguards needed. The patient needs help; the doctor tries out a procedure cautiously, remaining equally attentive to his patient's well-being and the advancement of knowledge.

Non-Therapeutic Research

Rutstein and Galabresi's procedures would more appropriately safeguard another kind of experimentation where often the subject of the experiment is not ill, the investigator is not a physician, and the experiment requires many subjects, perhaps thousands, to provide the necessary statistical data for analysis. The AMA defines non-therapeutic research as "clinical investigation primarily for the accumulation of knowledge." It would include the landmark experiments that Cotton Mather and Zabdiel Boylston carried out in Boston in the eighteenth century when they vaccinated some eight hundred people with cowpox vaccine as a prophylactic against smallpox, Salk's experiments with poliomyelitis vaccines on thousands of subjects, and the tests the Army carried out in the early part of this century on soldier-volunteers to see whether mosquitoes carried malaria. Even though the first two cases promised to benefit their subjects if they were successful, all three needed healthy people willing to run a risk in trying out a new medical procedure that could reduce the more remote risk that they could contract the disease in question.[8] In cases such as these, lacking the glue of the doctor-patient relationship, science and ethics are more likely to come unstuck. In the gap, an ambitious desire to triumph over competing experimenters working with a similar procedure could bring the physician-experimenter to treat his human subjects, especially if they are poor or institutionalized, as little more than guinea pigs. It has happened, as M. H. Pappworth's oft-cited <u>Human Guinea Pigs</u> (Boston: Beacon Press, 1968) attests.

The Need for Consent

Paul Ramsey, musing on the history of abuse documented in
Pappworth and in the Nuremburg trial cases of Nazi doctors,
writes:

> The likelihood that a researcher would make a mistake in de-
> parting from a generally valuable rule of medical practice be-
> cause he is biased toward the research benefits of permitting
> an "exception" is exceedingly great.... In the grand moral
> matters of life and death, of maiming or curing, of the violation
> of persons or their bodily integrity, a physician or experimenter
> is more liable to make an error in moral judgement if he adopts
> a policy of holding himself open to the possibility that there
> may be significant, future permissions to ignore the principle
> of consent than he is if he holds this requirement of informed
> consent always relevant and applicable.... Man's capacity to
> become joint adventurers in a common cause makes the con-
> sensual relation possible; man's propensity to overreach his
> joint adventurer even in a good course makes consent necessary.[9]

Ramsey would make non-therapeutic experimentation resemble
therapeutic experimentation as closely as possible by requiring
the experimenter to win a full and honest consent from the subjects of the experiment; they now have much less than self interest in their own health to motivate them. The experimenter's
respect for his subject must be a close equivalent to the respect
the physician has for his patient. Conversely, the subject must
be permitted to become an active participant in the experiment.

With a like mind, Margaret Mead, while admitting that wide-
scale experiments in large urban hospitals make a high level of
participation between experimenter and subject difficult, nevertheless insists that it is not impossible:

> But I submit that the intense willingness of an individual of any
> level of education to participate in an enterprise--because he
> himself is suffering, has suffered, or may suffer, because he
> himself is dignified by an order of social participation not
> readily available to him, or because, being intellectually alert,
> he is given a part in an intellectually stimulating exercise--is
> related to the degree of the involvement of the subject. Because
> he is personally involved through his experience, his fears, his
> solitude, his desire for recognition as a socially valuable per-

son, or his satisfaction in using his mind, he is by any one or
all of these routes removed from the demanding status of <u>guinea
pig</u>. Guinea pigs are not able to invoke their experience or
fears or cognitive powers in this way. These are distinctively
human and noble aspects of humanity....
We can further adopt the position that the failure to do research,
to experiment, and to learn is reprehensible. We can cease to
try to limit and curtail experiments on human beings, while we
devise more and better experiments <u>with</u> human beings who,
as participants, are collaborators.[10]

The Elusiveness of Consent

But true consent, it is almost universally acknowledged, is
devilishly hard to win. Even in therapeutic experimentation
the patient often does not or cannot fully understand the procedures to be tried, or the risks involved. The awed respect a
patient has for a physician can cloud the assessment of whether
the risk the physician asks the patient to take is worth it.
Furthermore, in non-therapeutic experiments with large numbers of subjects, the consent procedure often becomes routin-
ized, and with it comes pressure on, for example, the parents
of school children to be immunized against poliomyelitis, to go
along with the prevailing practice. The danger of manipulated
consent increases even more in institutional settings. Inmates
of public hospitals, mental wards, prisons, members of the
armed services, or students in a research-professor's
seminar can be very susceptible to what Edmond Cahn calls
"engineered consent":

> One of the major malpractices of our era consists in the "en-
> gineering of consent. " Sometimes this is effected simply by
> exploiting the condition of necessitious men as in certain In-
> dian states were thousands of consents to sexual sterilization
> have been purchased by offering a trivial bounty to the members
> of the destitute caste. Then again, consent may be "engineered"
> by the kind of psychologist who takes it for granted that his
> assistants and students will submit to experiments and implies
> a threat to advancement if they raise questions. Or the total
> community may "engineer" a consent, as when the president,
> the generals, and the newspapers call with loud fanfare for a
> heroic crew of astronautical volunteers to attempt some ultra-
> hazardous exploit.[11]

Restrictive Views of Consent

One response to the elusiveness of truly free consent is to
expect it to be infrequent. Hans Jonas makes a subtle analysis
of the social contract theory(according to which individuals
agree to limit their freedoms somewhat for the common good)
to show that medical experimentation with healthy human subjects is a unique case with its own special problems. To balance
individual freedom and societal needs in this case is very tricky
indeed. Primarily he says that restrictions on individual freedom are accepted not for the general common good, but because of the good that accrues to the individual in a society
where the common lot respects each other's inviolability.
Each of us who obeys a traffic light, pays taxes, or refrains
from yelling "fire" when there is none in a crowded theater
does so because it is for our own good if society as a whole
behaves in expected ways. Only in time of war, Jonas says,
is the social contract abrogated temporarily as a dispropor-
tionate burden is placed on one part of the population: the
young men who actually go to the front. Medical experimentation does not present an analogous case to war except in rare
epidemics where a whole society is treated in the same way it
would be by an enemy invasion. (Even the fight against cancer
is a fight against a disease that threatens only certain individuals in a society, not the society as a whole.) And because
volunteering for an experiment does not promise any immediate
good for the individual, it "falls somewhere between this over-
powering case and the normal transactions of the social contract."[12] Jonas concludes that society has no right to demand in
even the most subtle way that individuals sacrifice themselves
for medical experiments if there is no epidemic. Society rather
must depend on the "gracefulness" of utterly uncompelled
individuals to sacrifice their freedom or well-being at their
own pace:

> The destination of research is essentially melioristic. It does
> not serve the preservation of the existing good from which I
> profit myself and to which I am obligated. Unless the present
> state is intolerable, the melioristic goal is in a sense gratu-
> itous, and not only from the vantage point of the present. Our

descendants have a right to be left an unplundered planet; they
do not have a right to new miracle cures.... Progress, with
all our methodical labor for it, cannot be budgeted in advance
and its fruit received as a due. Its coming about at all and its
turning out for the good (of which we can never be sure) must
rather be regarded as something akin to grace. [13]

What Jonas means by "grace" becomes clearer when he describes those most likely to have it in volunteering for a non-
therapeutic experiment. The researcher's first subject should
be himself, Jonas says; then he or she should look for additional
subjects where a maximum of identification, understanding, and
spontaneity can be expected--among the highly motivated, the
educated, and least captive members of society (that is to say,
among other research scientists, or people with the training,
intelligence, and wisdom to really understand what a medical
investigator is up to). "Grace" is noblesse oblige. "The poorer
in knowledge, motivation, and freedom of decision (and that
alas means the more readily available in terms of numbers and
possible manipulation), the more sparingly and indeed reluc-
tantly should the reservoir be used, and the more compelling
must therefore become the countervailing justification."[14] Jonas
acknowledges that his stiff criterion would slow progress. This
is a price he thinks society should be willing to pay "for the
preservation of the most precious capital of higher communal
life."[15]

According to other writers who think like Jonas, such a
criterion would do more than slow progress. It would preserve the process of individual choice in a society that can
never improve upon it, for all the other progress of which it is
capable. Paul Ramsey would deny scientists access to children as subjects for non-therapeutic experiments. No one else
has the right to volunteer them if they can't mentally or legally
decide for themselves. The argument that a parent could
reasonably presume that the child would consent if it could
ignores the child's right to act unreasonably. Proxy consent
is not consent. He states categorically: "No one ought to
consent for a child to be made the subject of medical inves-
tigations primarily for the accumulation of scientific knowledge, except in the face of epidemic conditions that bring upon

the individual child disproportionately the same or likely
greater dangers. "16 Alvin Bronstein thinks along similar lines
when he says that prisoners cannot freely consent:

> My position with respect to the use of prisoners in non-thera-
> peutic medical experimentation is simple and clear; the de
> facto environment of prisons is such that you cannot create an
> institution in which informed consent without coercion is feas-
> ible. Given the nature of the institution of prisons, and the
> degree of intrusion on the individual, his body and his mind,
> which necessarily results from non-therapeutic medical ex-
> perimentation, the constitutional rights of the individual pris-
> oner to be free from invasions of privacy, free from invasions
> of his human dignity, free from cruel and unusual punishment,
> and free from injurious state action without due process are
> violated.17

More Permissive Views on Consent

Another response to the problem of imperfect consent is to
argue that the benefits to society from improved medical knowledge go a long way to forgive it. People usually aren't expected to give a perfect consent when their land is taken away
for a public highway. Young men do not freely consent to
military conscription. People could be encouraged to volunteer
for medical experiments by a government that could assess the
risks, monitor the experiments, and do all it could to reduce
the risk individuals take for the common good. Government,
in short, could share the burden of consent. Guido Galabresi
calls for procedures to strike a balance between individual
freedom and the common good in medical experiments:

> On the one hand, we want decisions that reflect societal choices
> and societal control when victims are taken for the common
> good. On the other hand, we do not want society to lose its
> role of protector of individual lives. These desires conflict,
> but both are essential to a decent society. Areas other than
> medical experimentation have managed more or less adequately
> to accommodate these conflicting needs. So far, medical
> experimentation has hardly tried. Consent, though useful in
> preserving the ideal that society hardly ever condones the

sacrifice of an individual against his will, is unlikely to suffice
where a too obvious societal choice to take victims is involved.
Even more important, consent cannot serve as the general control system determining when the future good requires the taking of present lives. Accordingly, scholars seriously concerned
with the problem of saving future lives and at the same time
not undermining our commitment to the sanctity of individual
present lives ought to be devoting themselves to the development of a workable but not too obvious control system, rather
than to the spinning-out of theories of consent. [18]

William J. Curran and Henry K. Beecher review the medical
codes in Britain and America pertaining to experimentation
with children. They suggest their own practical standards:
When the research is therapeutic for the good of the minor patient then he or she should be included in the study as long as
informed consent is obtained from the parents or guardian;
when the research is not therapeutic, subjects who are minors
fourteen years or older and intelligent enough to understand the
purposes, possible benefits, and hazards of the experiment
should be permitted to consent if their parents or guardians
consent as well. They conclude:

> There should be strong reasons in professional judgment
> for the use of immature children (those under 14 years of age)
> in any clinical investigation where there is no direct benefit
> intended for the child. However, such involvement should not
> be ruled out as illegal and unethical in all circumstances. Nei-
> ther American nor English law demands such a flat and sweep-
> ing condemnation. Such involvement should be allowed where
> the study has firm medical support and justification, promises
> important new knowledge of benefit to science and to mankind,
> and where there is no discernible risk involved for the child-
> subject. Not to allow such studies would greatly hamper im-
> portant nutritional, psychological, and educational studies in
> children as well as studies of inborn errors of metabolism and
> genetic defects. It should be noted also that studies in this
> category, involving no discernible risk, can be potentially, and
> sometimes unexpectedly, of direct benefit to a given subject.[19]

Louis Lasagna points out that for prisoners, participation in
experiments relieves boredom, and provides opportunities to
develop a sense of personal value. He reviews favorably the

non-therapeutic experiments carried out at Willowbrook State
School for the mentally retarded in New York, in which newly
admitted children were infected with a strain of hepatitis prevalent in the school in order to see whether or not immunity
could be acquired with a minimal experience of the disease. He
says that the procedure of inflicting unsuspecting children with
a disease might at first glance seem abhorrent, but that the
circumstances justified the experiment. Everyone admitted to
the school develops hepatitis anyway; in the experiment the
dosage could be adjusted to discover the precise minimum
needed to confer immunity, the experimental group was housed
separately, the protocol was reviewed and approved by several
agencies, and informed consent was obtained from the parents.[20]
(Paul Ramsey discusses the same experiment in Patient as Person and castigates it.[21]) Lasagna argues as a situation-ethician
that standards should be flexible, adaptable to the situation.
"It would seem preferable to avoid dogma, codes, pontifical
stands, and the temptation to talk in capital letters about THE
SANCTITY OF LIFE with the letters written with stars between
them, à la Hyman Kaplan."[22]

Geoffrey Edsall moreover suggests that there are certain
situations in which a decision not to allow subjects to be part
of an experiment might be, if not unethical, the cause of harm.
Initially the oral poliomyelitis vaccine carried a risk of infect-
ing one adult in a million with polio Type 3. One country which
decided on that basis not to permit use of the drug suffered a
much larger epidemic of Type 3 than the drug would have
caused. [23] Thinkers such as Curran, Beecher, Lasagna, and
Edsall can point to the practical benefits of large scale non-
therapeutic research with subjects whose consent has been less
than complete, but who nonetheless have gained a certain dignity
through their contributions. Jonas, Ramsey, and Bronstein
would consider any benefits dubious that were not rooted in the
free decisions of capable citizens. They fear dehumanization,
however efficient.

Fetal Research

Legal abortions daily produce a whole new medical entity:
living creatures doomed to die at a predictable time a few mo-

ments after being severed from their mother's life support system. The new laws permitting abortion seem to imply that the fetus is morally and legally less than human, for all its physiological resemblance to human life. Could experiments be done on fetuses doomed to die anyway that might enhance the chances of wanted fetuses to survive the perils of fetal life? To plot a course through this question certain distinctions become critical. A <u>nonviable</u> fetus, usually less than twenty-four weeks old and weighing less than eight hundred grams, is not expected to be able to live independently of its mother's body. It can be legally aborted. A <u>viable</u> fetus on the other hand might be able to live independently. It is legally protected against abortion, and should one be born inadvertently of the abortion process, it becomes legally a child which the attending physician is duty-bound to save whatever the mother's feeling for it. So experiments with a viable fetus would fall under the same guidelines as experiments with children; the proxy consent of the parents or the guardians of the child would have to be obtained. An equally basic distinction is made between a fetus, viable or nonviable, <u>in utero</u> or <u>ex utero.</u>

Most ethicians would agree that living tissue from a dead, legally aborted fetus <u>ex utero</u> is suitable for experimentation provided the mother or the parents assent to its use. And most would also agree that therapeutic experimentation <u>in utero</u> carried on for the benefit of either the nonviable or viable fetus or the mother would be laudable, provided the normal conditions were met for therapeutic experimentation with children or consenting adults. (The recently published report of the National Commission for the Protection of Human Subjects of Biomedical and Behavioral Research, considered below, takes these views.) Ethical debate centers on the availability for non-therapeutic experimentation of the nonviable, unwanted fetus alive <u>in utero</u> prior to a planned abortion, or dying immediately afterwards <u>ex utero.</u> The positions in the debate depend greatly on different ideas of how human a fetus is.

The Fetus as Tissue

Joseph Fletcher believes the previable fetus to be less than human:

Common sense...does not allow that a fetus which is nonviable or to be terminated can be "harmed" or "injured" or
"insulted, " since acts of battery and mayhem pre-suppose a living, independent individual biologically. Invasive treatment
of a fetus, in either therapy or experimentation, might come
under the heading in law of mutilation, as of a corpse, but
would not be an injury (injure or injustice). An injustice predi-
cates a person. The only injury could be to the maternal patient, and with the appropriate consent even that becomes null.24

Fletcher argues from this position that the fetus should be
considered expendable for any type of research "if it yielded
the medical knowledge wherewith to help many other fetuses,
live children, and adults. "25

Gary L. Rebach finds there is some legal basis for a position like Fletcher's. After reviewing the state and federal laws
regulating fetal research and finding them to be uncertain about
the nature of the nonviable fetus, it is his opinion that it would
be fair to treat a nonviable fetus as part of the mother: "...a
nonviable aborted fetus would be treated as a collection of the
mother's tissue, while experimentation on a nonviable fetus in
utero would be considered merely experimentation on the mother. Such a result may be medically logical; since an aborted
nonviable fetus cannot by definition develop into a normal infant, it is unclear that such a fetus should be treated as anything other than a collection of tissue for consent purposes. "26
Rebach acknowledges that this idea may be repugnant to many
because of the similarity of aborted fetuses to mature infants,
yet he feels it ethical and consistent with current legal standards.

The Fetus as a Child

Other writers consider the fetus as a child for whom the
mother can give proxy consent--but only for unharmful experiments. Leroy Walters argues that fetuses to be aborted should
be treated in the same way as fetuses to be brought to term;
no drastic experiments should be permitted on either. This
procedure would assure that the unwanted fetus was not crippled
in the womb. It would guard against the brutalization of the
experimenter who would be less likely to have experience treat-

ing human life even in its most primitive form as subhuman.
It would also permit a woman to make a last-minute decision
not to have an abortion; she wouldn't have the added pressure
to go through with an abortion from the likelihood that she was
carrying a medically mutilated fetus.[27]

Richard Wasserstrom believes that the fetus enjoys a unique
moral status, resting largely on its potential to become a fully
adult human being. When an abortion destroys this potential,
"then experimentation upon the fetus in no way affects the fetus'
ability or lack thereof, ever to realize any of its existing potential. On this view especially, abortion, not experimentation
upon the non-viable fetus, is the fundamental, morally problematic activity. "[28] He finds that only if it can be granted that
the morality of abortion is not in question can he somewhat reluc-
tantly conclude that experimentation on a dying fetus ex utero
may be permissible provided that the mother consents, that the
experiment is important, and that those medical persons who
counsel a woman concerning abortion should not be the same
persons involved in the experimentation.

Paul Ramsey takes the view that because the fetus's consent
for any non-therapeutic experimentation upon its person is indispensable and unobtainable, no non-therapeutic experiments
can be performed on it. He disallows proxy consent. He coun-
ters the argument that the evil of abortion can be mollified by
the evil of fetal research (so that some good could come of the
procedure) by saying simply that two wrongs do not make a
right. He disapproves of any determination "to wrest by our
scientific works some good out of guilt laden harmfulness to
unborn life. " [29]

The Commission on the Protection
of Human Subjects

The opinions of Fletcher, Walters, and Wasserstrom were
included in the report of the Department of Health, Education
and Welfare's Commission on the Protection of Human Subjects.[30]
The report summarizes a world-wide literature search on the
subject, establishes key definitions, reviews in detail four test
cases of experiments done on fetuses, reviews the positions of

its own commissioners whose opinions vary considerably,
makes its own recommendations for procedures that would have
to be followed in order for researchers to receive department
funding, and appends several dissents to its own recommendations. In its general conclusion, the commission basically
adopts the position that Walters developed: experiments can be
performed on fetuses in utero provided that fetuses to be aborted
are treated as if they were to be brought to term. Only no-
risk or minimal-risk experiments can be performed. A review
board is to determine in each case what constitutes "minimal
risk."

The commission states that the status of the nonviable,
dying fetus ex utero alters the situation in two ways:

> First, the question of risk becomes less relevant, since the
> dying fetus cannot be "harmed" in the sense of "injured for
> life." Once the abortion procedure has begun, or after it is
> completed, there is no chance of a change of mind on the woman's
> part which will result in a living injured subject. Second,
> however, while the questions of risk become less relevant, con-
> siderations of respect for the dignity of the fetus continue to
> be of paramount importance, and require that the fetus be treated
> with the respect due to dying subjects. While dying subjects
> may not be "harmed" in the sense of "injured for life," issues
> of violation of integrity are nonetheless central. The Commis-
> sion concludes, therefore, that out of respect for the dying sub-
> ject, no non-therapeutic interventions are permissible which
> would alter the duration of life of the non-viable fetus ex utero.[31]
> (Emphasis added)

Casper Weinberger, then secretary of the Department of
Health, Education and Welfare, however, qualifies the last
recommendation in his commentary on the report. He rules
that certain kinds of research will be permitted to alter the
duration of the life of the dying fetus:

> ...the Secretary is persuaded by the weight of scientific evi-
> dence that research performed on the non-viable fetus ex utero
> has contributed substantially to the ability of physicians to
> bring to viability increasingly small fetuses. The Secretary
> perceives that it is in the public interest to continue this
> successful research and accordingly an exception is made to

the Recommendations of the Commission to permit research to develop new methods for enabling fetuses to survive to the point of viability.[32]

Paul Ramsey dissents most vigorously from Weinberger's position. He comments extensively on its earlier forms in the two drafts of this report published in the Federal Register of 16 November 1973 and 31 August 1974 in his book, The Ethics of Fetal Research, published early in 1975. (In the earlier drafts the commission has permitted experimentations to alter the duration of life; the final draft withheld the permission, only to have the secretary reinstate it.)

Ramsey points out the irony that as the benefit to the individual fetus experimented upon would increase (as the unwanted fetus would approach salvageability with the techniques of the experiment), the experiment would have to be curtailed, lest the unwanted fetus lived. "That reverses the ordinary canons of medical ethics," he says flatly. "The closer such experiments come to being life saving or beneficial to the subject, the clearer it becomes that the use of still-living fetuses who could not possibly benefit and who might even be harmed by the trial was wrong in the first place." [33]

Chapter 2

Genetic Counseling and Screening

The Cases

1   A young married couple's first child is born with hemophilia, a sex-linked hereditary condition affecting almost exclusively males in which the blood fails to clot quickly enough,
causing prolonged uncontrollable bleeding from even the smallest cut. Their physician suggests they consult a genetic counselor about the possibilities that future children might be
afflicted with the same disease. A female fetus might carry
the gene that causes the disease but would not suffer from it.

Later the woman becomes pregnant and returns again
to the counselor for advice. He suggests she undergo amniocentesis to discover whether the fetus is male. In this procedure the uterus is perforated and amniotic fluid removed
from which the genetic makeup of the fetus can be analyzed.
The test cannot detect the disease, in this case, only the sex
of the fetus. It is male. The counselor informs the mother
again that there is a 50 percent chance the child is afflicted.
He intimates that she should have an abortion rather than run
the risk, suggesting that later she can try to conceive a healthy
infant. She follows his advice.

2   The parents of five girls have tried for several years to
give birth to a boy. But they decide after the mother reaches
the age of thirty-five not to have any more children because
of the high risk which a mother of that age runs of bearing a
child with Down's syndrome (formerly called mongolism, a
term now discouraged because of its misleading racial connota-
tion). When the woman inadvertently becomes pregnant again
at age forty, the couple approaches their family physician for
counseling. He advises amniocentesis; if the test is positive

they can abort the child. They agree. The test is negative.
The fetus appears to be very healthy. The parents are greatly
relieved.

From the test results, however, the physician has also
learned that the fetus is another girl. Because both parents
were committed to aborting a mongoloid fetus, and the physician knows from long acquaintance that both have long wanted a
boy, he fears that they might decide to abort a fetus known to
be a female. He decides not to tell them about its sex. He
thinks to himself that he in conscience could not be party to an
abortion for such trivial reasons.

3 A major clinic discovers a screening or testing procedure
for detecting Huntington's Chorea, a chronic disease which usually
manifests its symptoms in patients in middle age. At first
it causes involuntary jerking movements and eventually causes
the whole muscular system to deteriorate, resulting in gradual
paralysis and death. The tragedy of this presently incurable
disease is heightened by its manifesting its symptoms only long
after the victim has had children of his or her own. Half the
offspring of an afflicted parent will likewise be afflicted. The
screening tests the children of victims of the disease before
the children reach childbearing age. Twenty children are
screened in the first experiment. Seven are told that they will
have the disease, and must seriously consider whether to have
children of their own. The thirteen who are told they do not
have the disease are greatly relieved; two of the seven who do
commit suicide shortly afterwards.

Genetic Counseling: The Issues

In recent years when a woman has previously borne a child
with a genetic disease (a birth defect) such as albinism or
Down's syndrome, or when prospective parents know of
relatives on either side who have been afflicted with inherited
genetic diseases, they have often gone to seek the advice
of a genetic counselor. Trained in genetics, statistics,
and counseling, a counselor can develop a family tree with the
help of the parents to work out the odds that they will conceive
an afflicted child. He can arrange tests to analyze their

chromosomes. If the woman is already pregnant, the counselor
can arrange for the woman to undergo amniocentesis to probe
the genetic makeup of the fetus; if it is afflicted, the counselor
can help with the decision whether or not to abort.

Several recent developments have come together to make
counseling popular: contraception technology is now well enough
developed that a woman has a good chance of avoiding an unwanted pregnancy; there has been a great advance in the science
of genetics and the understanding of genetic disease; amniocentesis is now available; the Supreme Court has made abortion
a legal solution to an unwanted pregnancy.

The counselor must command broad scientific expertise as
well as a human sensibility. He or she must know the pathology
and possibilities for treatment of several hundred diseases and
be able to work out statistical probabilities or read the results
of chromosome or amniocentesis tests. The counselor is likely
to face people who are very nervous about bearing a diseased
child (perhaps they are already living with the strain of raising
one) or who often feel very guilty about what they have come to
think of as their "bad genes. " They might be facing for the
first time in their lives a serious personal decision--whether
or not to have an abortion. Beyond this, the counselor might
find the clients are making a decision with which he or she does
not agree personally, making it very difficult to remain neutral.
In the course of testing, the counselor might have discovered
that a woman's husband cannot possibly be the genetic father of
her fetus, or that one or another of the parents is afflicted
with a genetic disease whose symptoms haven't yet become
manifest. The counselor needs to be careful about how he or
she talks to the clients and about what is said.

The most difficult feature of counseling for both the clients
and the counselor (and the ethicians) is that while genetic diseases can be tested for, only a few can be cured. Detecting a
disease usually leads either to a decision to bear an afflicted
child or to abort an afflicted fetus. Abortion is obviously not
therapy for the fetus, only a possible consolation for the parents
--giving them another chance to conceive a healthy infant--and
so doctoring seems to be turned on its head: the patient is
abandoned in order to treat the effect its living would have on

others. Even more problematic is the chance with each testing
that a mistake will be made and a healthy fetus will die.

The Language of Genetics

Understanding a little about the science of genetics and its
application to genetic counseling can help in understanding the
discussion about its ethics. We can imagine that a counselor
might begin a counseling session with a description of the genetic structure inherent in every human cell.

All living cells in the human body contain molecules of DNA:
deoxyribonucleic acid. These long, very thin, cylindrical
molecules, if expanded to scale, would resemble a spaghetti
noodle twenty miles long. DNA molecules are made of four
chemical constituents comprising a genetic code which carries
the information determining the tens of thousands of chemical
reactions that make the body work, from the reactions that color
the eyes to those that build up the intricate structures of the
brain and other major organs. Every cell in the human body
carries the genetic code for the whole body.

The four chemical constituents that constitute DNA are known
as adenine (A), cytosine (C), guanine (G), and thymine (T). The
varied pattern of these constituents along a DNA molecule com-
prises a sort of four-letter alphabet; thus the genetic information
in DNA is arranged much like verbal information on a ticker
tape. A small segment of this tape--a gene--contains about
a thousand "letters." A typical gene "word" containing the
information that orders the cell to carry out one chemical reaction might look like this: TACCGGCTAATGTACAATGAGAGG,
and so on. A normal human cell contains tens of thousands of
such genes.

DNA in human cells is organized into forty-six packages
called chromosomes arranged in twenty-three identical-looking
pairs. (Each chromosome contains very roughly a thousand
genes.) Just prior to the division of a body cell into two cells,
each chromosome is replicated--an exact copy is produced.
Then, as the cell divides, each chromosome and its copy are
separated from one another; the original chromosome ends up
in one of the cells formed by division, the copy in the other.

In this way genetic information is passed intact from cell generation to cell generation in the cells that make up the body.

A special type of cell division occurs during the formation of a sperm or egg, however. In this case the pair of chromosomes become aligned side-by-side, gene-for-gene, and then replicate. This is followed by two cell divisions: the first one separates the chromosomes in a pair from each other, consigning one to each of the cells formed by the first division; the second division separates a chromosome from its copy, the original chromosome ending up in one cell, the copy in the other. The upshot of this special type of division is that each sperm or egg contains only twenty-three chromosomes--one of each type--not forty-six. In this state they are ripe for mating.

Sometimes, especially during a cell division when the chromosomes reduplicate themselves, a "misprint" can occur so that the sequence of letters in a chromosome becomes aberrant. This creates a "mutation." The new aberrant information in the chromosome, if followed, could cause an abnormal chemical reaction to take place someplace in the body with possibly catastrophic results. In one example, the body might not be able to oxidize phenylpyruvic acid in the central nervous system, thus causing severe mental deficiency; this disease is called PKU or phenylketonuria.

Usually when a gene is defective, the defect doesn't have any effect at all. The healthy partner gene on the other chromosome of the pair carries on the work. The mutant gene is said to be recessive. But occasionally, the abnormal gene is so powerful that it overwhelms the effects of the normal gene. The abnormality is then said to be dominant. Such defects are very rare and usually serious. Those afflicted rarely live long enough to reproduce themselves and their abnormal chemistry.

More frequently, birth defects occur when a defective gene (caused by a mutation long ago in the genes of a remote ancestor) in a father's sperm matches up with an identical defective gene in the mother's egg at conception. Then only wrong information can be sent by the paired genes. It has been estimated that everyone carries between three and eight defective genes; their pairing up with identical defective genes occurs only rarely, however, because everyone has very different ones. None-theless, each human being is a walking arsenal of destructive genes that are passed from generation to generation until finally and perhaps inevitably their power to harm emerges.

Working Out Probabilities

Having said this, the counselor might then help the prospective parents to assess the likelihood of their producing a child with an abnormal gene pairing. He or she would with their help trace through their family trees for any pattern of a recurring genetic disease to assess whether either one of them might have inherited recessive genes for it. If a pattern appears, he or she might explain that it occurred (and might continue) as a consequence of the special type of cell division giving rise to sperm and eggs. If a father carries a mutant gene on one chromosome of a pair, and a normal gene on the other, then half the sperm he produces will carry the mutant gene and the other half will carry the normal gene. If the mother also carries a normal and a mutant gene, half the eggs will carry the mutant, and half the normal gene. At fertilization, the sperm and egg join at random. In any conception of the sperm and egg of two carrier parents, there is one chance in four that both mutant genes will come together and two chances in four that a normal gene will come together with a mutant one.

The counselor would tell the prospective parents that on the average the same distribution would hold for four children born to any number of parents who are recessive carriers. Four sets of parents bearing one child each would tend to produce the same ratio of afflicted children, carriers, and normals. And the odds would be the same for each of the subsequent children they would bear. It's possible that by a twist of fate all their children will be free of the defective gene completely, or that all will be afflicted.

One important exception to the rules of inheritance should be noted: the process and the odds work somewhat differently with sex-linked disorders such as hemophilia and the relatively common and harmless red-green colorblindness. Many genes causing genetic diseases are sex-linked; that is, they are carried on the chromosomes that determine sex. Normal males have in addition to twenty-two pairs of identical-looking chromosomes, one pair in which the chromosomes do not match in shape and size. These are the sex-chromosomes; the longer of the pair is called the X-chromosome, the shorter, the Y-chromosome. The Y-chromosome in humans and many other organisms seems to carry very few genes other than those that trigger male development in the embryo. The X-chromosome, on the other hand, carries many genes; these are known as sex-linked genes.

Normal females carry two X-chromosomes in addition to twenty-two other pairs; thus, they carry twenty-three pairs of chromosomes altogether. In the formation of eggs, the X-chromosomes (and the other chromosomes as well) become separated from their partners; the egg therefore carries twenty-three chromosomes, one X-chromosome and one of each of the other twenty-two types. In males, during the formation of sperm, the X and the Y become separated. Half the sperm will carry one X-chromosome plus one of each of the other twenty-two types; half will carry the Y along with one of each of the other twenty-two types. When the egg and the sperm unite at fertilization, half the fertilized eggs will receive two X's plus twenty-two pairs of other chromosomes (and will therefore be female); the other half will receive an X and a Y plus twenty-two pairs of other chromosomes (and therefore be male).

Because of this pattern of inheritance, a recessive mutation on the X-chromosome in a male offspring will be expressed; the mutation has no normal partner on the Y to conceal its effects. Thus a female carrying a normal gene at some position of one of her X-chromosomes will transmit it to half her sons and they will be normal, and the mutant gene on the other X to the other half of her sons, and they will be affected. An affected male, on the other hand, can transmit his mutation-bearing X only to his daughters. Since the daughters will almost always receive a non-mutant X from their mother, they will not be affected, although they will be carriers of the mutation.

Certain abnormalities are due not to specific mutations, but to an abnormal number of chromosomes. Most fertilized eggs with an abnormal number of chromosomes undergo spontaneous abortion at some time during the pregnancy, usually very early. One exception--which affects about one in 650 newborn children-- is Down's syndrome. Children with one type of Down's syndrome have forty-six chromosomes plus an extra one. (For convenience, the chromosome pairs other than the X and Y have been assigned numbers from one to twenty-two; in the case of Down's syndrome, the extra chromosome is a number twenty-one--the smallest chromosome of the set.) Most cases of Down's syndrome arise from a mistake during sperm or egg production in one of the parents (usually the mother), and the abnormal sperm or egg contains two copies of chromosome twenty-one instead of only one. Most couples who have had a child with Down's syndrome have a rather low chance of producing another one. The risk, however, depends on the age of the mother and in some cases whether one of the parents carries a certain type of chromosome abnormality that predisposes them to a high risk of Down's syndrome among their children.

In any event, for many diseases whose inheritance is due to a single mutant gene and for most types of chromosome abnormality, if the parents have produced no afflicted children but come from families with histories of genetic illness the counselor can often work out the probability that the parents are carriers from an analysis of the family tree of each.

Screening the Unborn

The counseling session takes on a different moral dimension when the woman of a couple who are known or suspected carriers becomes pregnant and wonders whether she should bear the fetus to term. The counselor can work out the probabilities using the procedures described, and he or she can also counsel that the woman undergo amniocentesis after twelve to sixteen weeks of the pregnancy. It is only at this relatively late stage that the amniotic fluid in the uterus contains fetal cells which can be analyzed. In cases where the disease can be detected using fetal cells, the test usually indicates whether the child is afflicted, although there is some margin of error. The test results take about three weeks to analyze. If the woman decides to abort

an afflicted fetus, then she might be already in her eighteenth
week of pregnancy and thus risk a dangerous abortion.

It is clear that the counseling procedure could bring either
great relief or great anxiety to prospective parents. They can
learn that there is minimal risk of their bearing children with
a particular defect, or that a fetus in utero is healthy. Or they
can both be brought to face a difficult decision: whether to
have children at all, or to abort an afflicted fetus, or to live with
an afflicted child. If the amniocentesis is positive, there are
rarely any other alternatives. A few genetic diseases can be
treated--PKU with a low phenylalanine diet, diabetes with
insulin--but none can be completely cured with any current
technology.

Moral Dilemma in Genetics : The Stigma of Being a Carrier

Genetic counselors themselves admit that counseling sessions
are very disturbing ordeals for their clients. More often parents
contemplating or having already conceived a child come to a
counselor because of their real fear of bearing a defective child.
Genetic defects run in their family; a genetically defective child
has already been born to the mother. Because of their firsthand experience with the shock of the birth of such a child, and
the difficulty and expense of raising one, they want to be sure that
they will bear only normal children in the future. Guilt often
accompanies their fear. Genetic counselor F. Clarke Fraser
tells of an incident in which a teenage girl became a drug addict
after discovering through counseling that she was a carrier of a
genetic disease. She is typical, he says, of the many carriers
of lethal genes who interpret their genetic abnormality as a
moral stigma, proof given them by some higher power that they
are less than fully human.[1]

The Pressure to Abort

John Fletcher, a sociologist who has studied the practice of
counseling, points out that the counseling sessions themselves
often intensify the moral dilemma for the parents. "The struc-

ture of the counseling situation calls for a readiness to be committed to abortion as the means of managing a positive diagnosis...." But the parents are usually at the same time committed to having more children, if only normal ones. "Wanting another child (sometimes desperately) and being explicitly committed to abortion constitute a tension of severely conflicting loyalties and is perceived as a moral problem."[2]

The implicit commitment to abortion sends out other shock waves. Parents often feel ashamed of what the act of aborting a genetically deformed fetus says to a living child of theirs or a relative who already has the disease. "So, you'd rather have me dead?" is the imagined response. Some feel discomfort at the thought that they as parents are opting for a double standard. Fletcher reports that one father said he would choose abortion over another retarded child, yet realized "if the majority of people reasoned in a similar manner about all children, a 'tyranny of the majority' could develop, aided by an exclusive value on 'intelligence' and having little tolerance for weakness or sickness."[3] All but the most solid of marriages are seriously shaken by the strain, Fletcher says, especially while waiting for the results of amniocentesis to come in.

The Difficulty of Remaining Objective

The counselors who open their procedures to public scrutiny admit that they find remaining objective very difficult, but that they work very hard at it. Fraser writes,

> ...I find that I tend to take a very pragmatic view of the situation. I am not very good at seeing the broad ethical issues and consequences in an individual situation. I tend to try and work towards the best solution for the immediate family as I see it, and rarely if ever does this conflict with my own ethics or morals, such as they are.... If they push me about what I think they should do--sometimes they say, "Well, what would you do if you were in my situation?" and I say that I cannot really put myself in their situation because I am not like them. If I try to, as best I can, then I tell them I think I would not have a baby, or have one, as the case may be. But it is very difficult to be objective about this, and one must beware of projecting one's own personality into the situation."[4]

For all their sincerity and efforts at being objective, however, differing convictions about how the counseling practice should be run results in making it a very different procedure from clinic to clinic. Fletcher says that the policy at the counseling center he studied was not to require that parents agree beforehand to abort any fetus amniocentesis indicated to be defective. The aim of the clinic was to "sharpen alternatives" so that the parents could make the most informed decision. He acknowledges that this practice seems to be an exception from the prevailing practice. Arno G. Motulsky justifies the more prevalent approach in his clinic: "Interuterine diagnosis is usually not offered to parents unless they are willing to have an affected fetus aborted. For patients unwilling to take that step, diagnosis of a disease in a fetus would serve no useful purpose and would only create anxiety and grief to the parents. "[5]

Paul Ramsey thinks amniocentesis is itself morally questionable and so any style of counseling this procedure would be equally reprehensible. He thinks counselors have had to come to believe that their overriding goal is producing healthy children only to assuage their consciences about the jettisoning of unhealthy ones. Until now, he says, the major tenet of medical ethics has been that one individual is never interchangeable with another; amniocentesis leads to its violation.

Ramsey can morally justify screening for contagious diseases which threaten everyone including the person tested and against which remedies exist. He can justify screening as an extension of genetic counseling, having in view informed decision making about parenthood. But proxy consent to screen for noncontagious illnesses in unborn or newly born individuals is only justifiable if the objective is treatment and no harm is done by the test.

Intrauterine screening by amniocentesis he finds ethically most problematic. Statistics show 1 to 2 percent of the tests harm either the fetus or its mother; in the case of the fetus, the injury may be fatal. Some of those harmed are bound to be diseased individuals discarded so that healthy ones can take their place; others are bound to be healthy ones sacrificed for the greater good of knowing whom to abort among the surviving 98 percent. Ramsey finds even more problematic the case

of a woman carrying the gene for hemophilia deciding to abort
any fetus amniocentesis finds to be male. A healthy infant is
aborted half the time. Only by looking at numbers to argue in
terms of statistical morality (it's for the good of the greatest
number) or in terms of cost effectiveness (it's for producing
more productive children) can one justify sacrificing the innocent. "If they may be harmed, then to presume their consent
is a violent presumption, which would advance physical health
at the expense of the moral health of our society and of medical
practice."[6]

Another mark against amniocentesis for Ramsey is the fate
of false-positives--healthy fetuses thought to be afflicted--who
are occasionally aborted or given treatment that might harm
them. It has happened that a child falsely diagnosed as a PKU
baby was put on a low phenylalanine diet which had the same
effects on the healthy child that not going on the diet would
have had on a diseased child. There is a similar danger of a
false diagnosis in cases involving "blighted ova," or balanced
carriers. In a twin pregnancy, it can happen that one of the
fetuses is normal, the other afflicted with Down's syndrome.
Both develop to a certain point when the afflicted one dies, becoming what is known as a blighted ovum. If some of its cells
are drawn off in anmiocentesis, an abnormal fetus may be
suspected to inhabit the womb, and a healthy fetus aborted. A
fetus with a "balance chromosome" could be perfectly normal
and yet possess chromosomes detectable by amniocentesis
usually found only in severely retardeds. In both cases an
abortion could kill a healthy fetus paradoxically under the
auspices of producing greater numbers of healthy children.
Not knowing enough even after amniocentesis makes its use
morally problematic.[7]

The Right to Know

Other ethical problems arise in counseling from knowing
too much. A counselor can discover information very embarrassing or very difficult to explain to the clients. He or
she might be tempted to pass over it in silence. Phillip R.
Reilly, who studies the legal obligations of disclosure for

counselors, finds the most useful guidelines in a legal pre-
scription covering all types of doctor-patient relationships.

> A physician violates his duty to his patient and subjects
> himself to liability if he withholds any facts which are neces-
> sary to form the basis of an intelligent consent by the patient
> to the proposed treatment. Likewise the physician may not
> minimize the known dangers of a procedure or operation in
> order to induce his patient's consent. At the same time, the
> physician must place the welfare of his patient above all else and
> this very fact places him in a position in which he sometimes
> must choose between two alternative courses of action. One is
> to explain to the patient every risk attendant upon any surgical
> procedure or operation, no matter how remote; this may well
> result in alarming a patient who is already unduly apprehensive
> and who may as a result refuse to undertake surgery in which
> there is in fact minimal risk; it may also result in actually in-
> creasing the risks by reason of the physiological result of the
> apprehension itself. The other is to recognize that each patient
> presents a separate problem, that the patient's mental and
> emotional condition is important and in certain cases may be
> crucial, and that in discussing the element of risk a certain
> amount of discretion must be employed consistent with the full
> disclosure of facts necessary to an informed consent.[8]

Reilly himself argues that the need for the family to make
its own decisions binds the genetic counselor to full disclosure,
even, he says, if the counselor finds it difficult to be neutral
about what he or she suspects its decision might be or if a
woman concerned only about bearing a Down's syndrome child is
discovered by amniocentesis to be carrying a fetus with another
milder disorder. But he leaves hanging the question whether
an amniocentesis which inferred that the husband of the fetus's
mother could not be its genetic father need be disclosed. Alexander Capron finds the discussion about disclosure reminiscent
of the early discussions of how much dying patients should be
told about their condition. The question in both situations, he
says, is not whether to tell, but how to tell; the best idea is
"beginning with the assumption that the information should be
conveyed and then applying one's creativity to devising a sensitive, humane means of conveying it. "[9]
A related problem is what a counselor should do with what he

or she learns about how a disease was transmitted through a
family's history. To trace a family tree, a counselor must pry
into the medical history of all the recent family members. Has
he or she the right, and is there corresponding obligation, to
tell other family members about their possible carrier status?
Reilly discovers that most laws dealing with medical practice
revere professional secrecy; presently there exists no code of
ethics precisely tuned to genetic counseling. He suggests that
in this ambiguous atmosphere it would probably be best to get
the client's consent to solicit or to relay information. A woman
who didn't want her family to know that she had conceived or
aborted a genetically diseased fetus might be able to sue the
doctor responsible for their finding out. A counselor might
have to endure the dilemma of protecting the privacy of a client while allowing other people obliviously to conceive diseased
infants. Similarly, if a family doesn't want a counselor to know
its history, a client's genetic load will have to be determined by
other, perhaps less efficient, means.

The Effect of Counseling
on the Future Human Life

The peculiar nature of genetic counseling is most apparent
when we see that the normally commendable dedication of a physician to a patient can, in genetic counseling, become distorted
into a dilemma as by a concave mirror. To understand how this
can happen, we need to consider how genetic counseling can
affect the health of future generations. Every mother who aborts
an afflicted fetus destroys with it two defective genes, and thus
seems to drain the pool of two genes for the next generation.
Usually, however, genetically afflicted children do not themselves grow up to bear children and so their defective genes
are not likely to be passed on by them anyway. Without an
afflicted child to care for, prospective parents tend to try to
conceive more non-afflicted or carrier children. The odds now
become two in three that each non-aborted, non-afflicted child
brought to term will be a carrier of one recessive defect. Thus,
paradoxically, abortions of genetically afflicted children tend to
encourage the births of an increased number of carriers, adding
to the steady trickle of mutations into the gene pool. Even if

the percentage of increase might be very slow, in the long run
more and more people would become carriers for a defect and
more and more likely to marry another carrier. Abortion might
become a common occurrence for producing a healthy family.

A similar effect results from the treatment of genetic ills.
Every diabetic on insulin treatment who can live a normal life
and have children insures the increase in the number of diabetics. If at any time in the future, maintenance technology fails,
all the afflicted offspring would have to pay the price at once.
Similarly, the slow increase in the number of carriers of genetic diseases dedicates or condemns future generations to develop the medical technology to cope with the problem. Herman
Muller envisions some point in the future when "the job of ministering to infirmities would come to consume all the energy
that society could muster for it, leaving no surplus for general,
cultural purposes."10

Most counselors aware of this dilemma opt for the present
needs of their living clients. Fraser writes:

> I try to follow the principle of acting for the good of the imme-
> diate family, so I do not bring the question of eugenics into the
> situation. Sometimes the parents do, however, and if so,
> I say to them that we really don't know enough about the things
> that control the frequencies of genes in populations to be able
> to say anything sensible about the eugenic aspects of their par-
> ticular action, and that their decision should be based on the
> future of their own children, rather than on considerations of
> posterity in general.11

James Crow, a geneticist, says that the future "can take care
of itself.... If we ask about the very long future, I would still
argue for humanitarian considerations in the current generation
on the grounds that we are learning more, and what we decide
to do that is wrong in this generation can be reversed in the next
generation if a wiser course of action becomes apparent."12

Another way of phrasing the question about the future effects
of modern genetic counseling is to ask whether by using it, human beings are subtly undermining traditional concepts of what
it means to be a human being. Along with an increased understanding of bad genes, is there a decrease in respect for the
"abnormal" individual? Is there less willingness to accept the

lot of all human beings, however sick or healthy? With this phrasing, the debate grows more philosophical and sharper.

Robert S. Morison, another counselor, sees nothing wrong with society's encouraging parents (without force) to make decisions to improve the lot of their offspring:

> If society has a definable and legitimate interest in the number of children to be born, then it is clear that it also may have an interest in the quality.... Now, when a defective child may cost the society many thousands of dollars a year for a whole lifetime without returning any benefit, it would appear inevitable that society should do what it reasonably can to assure that those who are born can lead normal and reasonably independent lives.... There is a limited number of slots that human beings can occupy, and there seem to be both social and family reasons to see that those increasingly rare slots are occupied by people with the greatest possible potential for themselves and for others.[13]

Fletcher, in summing up his study of the counseling procedure, suggests that today's parents and their society as well as the societies of the past and future have been and will continue to be engaged in an ongoing process of changing human nature: "...the most characteristic act of man is to attempt to change himself and his condition. Human freedom is an experiment in itself, conducted within the limits of human finitude and self interest."[14] He makes these remarks while speaking approvingly of the caution he has observed in the "consumers" of genetic progress. They use abortion only as a last resort to prevent bearing afflicted children. They had no interest in abortion for sex selection or for other trivial reasons. Change in their hands would be sure to be moderate, at pace with the developing technology and the changing identity of human life.

Other voices in the discussion are less optimistic and tend to argue from a less fluid concept of the nature of human beings. Daniel Callahan worries about the attitude we are going to take towards people afflicted permanently with genetic diseases while we go about the task of curing those patients who are curable. Are the chronic sick to become embarrassments? Perhaps the great distress parents feel now about living with an afflicted child or bearing one stems from their feeling that society is

blaming them for a failure. Societal pressure to bear only normal children could make it increasingly difficult to decide not
to abort a fetus suspected to be afflicted. Behind such pressure,
Callahan fears a developing standard of human perfectibility
that could be rather harshly applied to all sorts of less than perfect human beings. In the drive towards human perfectibility,
we could be retreating back to the standards of Sparta--the
Greek warrior state which threw all unhealthy looking babies off
a mountain cliff:

> We cure disease by ceasing to romanticize it, by gathering our
> powers to attack it, by making it an enemy to be captured. We
> learn to live with a disease, however, in a very different way:
> by trying to accept and cherish those who manifest the disease,
> by shaping social structures and institutions which will soften
> the individual suffering brought on by the disease, by refusing
> to make the bearer of the disease our economic, social, or
> political enemy. [15]

Leon Kass makes a systematic study of all the reasons
usually presented in defense of genetic abortion and rejects
every one. The first one he considers is the argument for the
good of society, which reasons that as society has an interest
in the genetic fitness of its members, it would be foolish to
waste precious resources caring for children who promise to
be unproductive. In response, Kass says that healthy children
cost a great deal as well: "Who is a greater drain on society's
precious resources, the average inmate of a home for the retarded, or the average graduate of Harvard College?"[16] Furthermore, he asks, how can "contribution" be assessed? He quotes
Pearl Buck on the subject of being a mother of a child retarded
by PKU:

> My child's life has not been meaningless. She has indeed
> brought comfort and practical help to many people who are
> parents of retarded children or are themselves handicapped.
> True, she has done it through me, yet without her I would not
> have had the means of learning how to accept the inevitable
> sorrow, and how to make that acceptance useful to others.
> Would I be so heartless as to say that it has been worthwhile
> for my child to be born retarded? Certainly not, but I am say-
> ing that even though gravely retarded it has been worthwhile
> for her to have lived.

It can be summed up, perhaps, by saying that in this world, where cruelty prevails in so many aspects of our life, I would not add the weight of choice to kill rather than to let live. A retarded child, a handicapped person, brings its own gift to life, even to the life of normal human beings. That gift is comprehended in the lessons of patience, understanding, and mercy, lessons which we all need to receive and to practice with one another, whatever we are.[17]

Another argument in favor of aborting genetically afflicted children is that it is for the good of the parents. This argument states that parents have a right to determine the quality of their family life, and that birth of a seriously defective child could cause great suffering for the normal children in the family. In response, Kass says that he respects the argument--one cannot presume to estimate for them how much of a burden an individual family can bear. But he says he isn't sure just what would be the best family life for healthy children to experience. Perhaps learning how to live with suffering graciously would make better people of us all. "Some have even speculated that the lack of experience with death and serious illness in our affluent young people is an important element in their difficulty in trying to find a way of life, and in responding patiently yet steadily to the serious problems of our society."[18] He is leery, he says, of the tendency to regard children as property for the pleasure of their parents.

Another argument is that persons who will suffer from a serious genetic disease won't be capable of living the full life of a human being anyhow. A giraffe with a short neck is not a giraffe; a child suffering from Down's syndrome is not a child. Nature itself causes many such afflicted fetuses to be spontaneously aborted or to die soon after birth. Induced abortion simply augments the tendency of nature to select naturally:

The advantages of this approach are clear. The standards are objective and in the fetus itself, thus avoiding the relativity and ambiguity in societal and parental good. The standard can be easily generalized to cover all such cases and will be resistant to the shifting sands of public opinion.
   This standard, I would suspect, is the one which most physicians and genetic counselors appeal to in their heart of

hearts, no matter what they say about letting the parents choose.
Why else would they have developed genetic counseling and
amniocentesis? [19]

The difficulty with this approach, Kass goes on to say, is that
the boundary line between the potentially human and potentially
inhuman is always going to be questionable. Genetic diseases
admit of varying degrees of severity. Who is to say which
diseases (congenital blindness? deafness? quadruplegia?) make
human life unlivable? "...It is the natural standard which may
be the most dangerous one in that it leads most directly to the
idea that there are second-class human beings and sub-human
beings."[20] Shades of Nazi eugenics arise.

Mass Genetic Screening: The Issues

During the early 1960s, scientists developed a simple, cheap,
and accurate test for PKU, requiring for analysis only a few
drops of blood from a newborn baby's heel. If a detected child
were put on a special diet of mushy pablum until it was four to
six years old, resisting every temptation to snitch a snack of
normal food, it could stave off mental retardation. Because
it was cheaper to screen all newborn babies for the disease
than to pay for the institutional care of the few who would be
afflicted, and because no one really could oppose any hopeful
therapy when it cost so little, almost every state makes
screening newborns for PKU mandatory.

As one blood or urine sample could serve for many tests, the
stage was set for screening for other genetic diseases as tests
for them became available. Since 1974, New York State has
been screening for PKU, sickle-cell anemia, maple syrup urine
disease, galactosemia, homocystinuria, adenosine deaminase
deficiency, and histidinemia. Other states have similar programs.

As genetic science developed in the 1960s, and as the public
became aware of genetic disease, adults in certain commu-
nities were urged to be screened for certain indigenous genetic
diseases. Eastern European Jews occasionally carry recessive genes for Tay-Sach's disease, a rare but fatal
disorder of an infant's nervous system. One of every ten black

Americans carries the "trait" or recessive gene for sickle-cell anemia, an ultimately fatal disease. The motive behind screening adults was alerting them to their possible carrier status so that they might seek out mates who didn't carry the recessive genes. If detected carriers were already married to each other, they could be urged to seek genetic counseling before bearing a child.

More recently, these mass genetic screening practices have become controversial. Paul Ramsey raises the issue of possible false-positive test results which could inflict the pablum diet on a healthy child and cripple it. Phillip Reilly points out that Rhode Island screens for maple syrup urine disease which has an incidence of only one in 300,000 births; a child with the disease is likely to be born in such a small state once in a decade. He suggested that we should rather screen for more common, treatable diseases. Some geneticists have called for a moratorium on screening until it can be examined by the whole community, fearing that screening programs aimed at minority groups could easily be perverted by some unscrupulous power into genocidal restrictions on reproduction.[21] Some ethicians see the danger that a biochemical abnormality "which is only a manifestation of normal genetic heterogeneity may initially be regarded as 'deviant.'"[22] In another place Marc Lappé warns of the deleterious side effects information about a person's genes could have on self-image. If an XYY baby boy is expected to develop into a criminal (after a controversial study found that a larger percentage of XYY males were found in prison populations than in the population at large) and is treated with suspicion, he just might do so. Insurance companies might deny coverage to carriers of various diseases. Worst of all, a carrier might come to hate himself or herself, assuming blame for "defects of nature" over which he or she has no control and which, ironically, aren't even detrimental to health.[23] Ramsey suggests that "in the face of the mounting genetic information, there may indeed be a 'right not to know,' if all of life's spontaneities are not to be toned down to the impersonal level of the laboratory or all of us learn to smell disease everywhere."[24]

Mandatory or Voluntary

The practical focus of the debate over screening is whether
it should be mandatory or voluntary. A screen is much easier
and more efficient if it is done routinely with no questions asked.
Patients or parents aren't likely to be scared off by lengthy
solicitations for their consent, or by their (from the screener's
point of view) unwarranted fears. In a letter to the editors of
The New England Journal of Medicine, five members of the
Task Force on Genetics and Reproduction at Yale, Subsection
on Heterozygous Carriers, wrote: "We believe that the right
of a newborn infant to intellectual development takes precedence
over the parent's right to allow or to refuse PKU screening for
their child. As we approach a period when in utero therapy
may prevent or minimize the effects of a genetic disease we
suggest that a diseased fetus has the right to optimal therapy.
This will often necessitate screening of the parents. "[25]

John A. Osmundsen thinks that screening should be routine
and comprehensive: Knowledge about genetic disorders can be
used to help reduce suffering; ease the economic cost of institutional care and the indirect costs of the loss of income of a
retarded child; help scientists to determine the precise health
needs of a society and to allocate resources for them; and
help families in improving the quality of their lives. He
adds "the bottom line in practically all instances where such
analyses have been made--for both the general population and
the high risk 'target' populations--is that screening saves
money, as well as despair, pain, and suffering. The estimated
cost of a malformed child is $250,000. According to figures
from the late 1950's there are about 250,000 defective births
annually in the United States alone--about 6% of all live births,
and 80% of those due wholly or partly to genetic factors. Think
about it. "[26]

Osmundsen dissents strongly from Paul Ramsey's notion
that mass screening is unethical because, as he sees Ramsey's
position, it "might abort a few perfect fetuses by mistake. " He
retorts that Ramsey ignores almost completely the person of
primary concern: "The defective patient with preventable
genetic disease. What about him?" [27] Osmundsen is arguing
against Ramsey in the course of a broader attack on the Report

from the Research Group on Ethical, Social, and Legal Issues
in Genetic Counseling and Genetic Engineering of the Institute
of Society, Ethics and the Life Sciences, of which Ramsey was
a member. Osmundsen seized on the report's major statement:
"There is currently no public health justification for mandatory
screening for the prevention of genetic disease. The conditions
being tested for in screening programs are neither contagious,
nor for the most part, susceptible to treatment at present."
He claims such a statement gives the institute the credibility
of the Flat Earth Society. He cites the treatments that are
available, and those that are being developed, as well as the
benefits to society that accrue from the systematic abortion
of identified uncurables.

Marc Lappé, the program director of the research group,
responds in the succeeding pages of the journal, saying
basically that Osmundsen misses the point of his citation and
the intent of the whole report. It proscribes mandatory
screening without denying the benefits that accompany risks of
voluntary screening. When taken up voluntarily, the risks of
screening become personal hazards by personal choice rather
than by legislative fiat. A summary of the report [28] follows:

--Screening programs should have specific goals, such as
the detection of a specific disorder, or the compilation of
disease distribution for a specific study. The purpose of the
programs should be to inform couples about the nature of
existing alternatives and potential therapies. Non-therapeutic
research should be linked to therapeutic counseling; whatever
information a study might discover that could be of use to
individual couples or persons must be made available to them.

--Screening programs designed to reduce the frequency of
carriers are unacceptable: "Virtually everyone carries a
small number of deleterious or lethal recessive genes, and to
reduce the frequency of a particular recessive gene to near the
level maintained by recurrent mutation, most or all persons
heterozygous for that gene would have either to refrain from
procreation entirely or to monitor all their off-spring in utero
and abort not only afflicted homozygote fetuses but also the
larger number of heterozygote carriers of the gene" (p. 243).

--Screening programs should be well planned, with quality review boards to assess the protocols. Programmers should take care to elicit community support for their screening; there should be equal access to the procedure for all who wished to be screened.

--Screening should have no strings attached: "As a general principle, we strongly urge that no screening program have policies that would in any way impose constraints on child-bearing by individuals of any specific genetic constitution, or would stigmatize couples who, with full knowledge of the genetic risks, still desire children of their own" (p. 245). Genetic diseases are to be clearly distinguished from contagious diseases which meance public health. "The conditions being tested for in a screening program are neither 'contagious' nor, for the most part, susceptible to treatment at present" (p. 245).

--Screening should be voluntary. "We seriously question the rationale of screening preschool minors or preadolescents for sickle-cell disease or trait since there is a substantial danger of stigmatization and little medical value in detecting the carrier state at this age" (p. 246).

--All the results of a screening should be given to the persons screened, no matter how complicated. Counseling should be made available for those found heterozygotes or homozygotes. "As a general rule, counseling should be non-directive, with an emphasis on informing the client and not making decisions for him" (p. 242). Under no circumstances should screening be construed as tacit acceptance of therapy or abortion.

--Researchers should protect screening information from being distributed irresponsibly. "...Misuse or misinterpretation must be seen as one of the principle potentially deleterious consequences of screening programs" (p. 248). Care should be taken to protect participants against stigmatization which could arise from making knowledge of a person's carrier status public in any way. Young children should not be recommended to refrain from physical activity because of carrying the sickle-cell trait; life-insurance coverage should not be denied adult trait carriers.

Screening for Huntington's Chorea: A Special Case

Screening for Huntington's Chorea creates a particularly poignant dilemma. Here the presently healthy seeming individuals who undergo the test might be found to carry the latent form of the disease itself, not merely the recessive gene, and may discover themselves doomed to suffer its hideous effects. Most of those screened have already seen a parent suffer from it; 50 percent of their children can also be expected to inherit the same fate; the test will let them know for certain into which division they fall. One writer responds "It is not unreasonable to withhold the use of a test of this sort until we have something tangible to offer those who give a positive result. "[29] Willard Gaylin takes a more moderate view. Mandatory screening is out of the question but: "The availability of such procedures should be widely and actively publicized. The usefulness of a medical procedure depends on its utilization, not its potential. To perfect a procedure and to keep this from public awareness because one assumes that the patient populations may not be able to tolerate the choice offered is a paternalistic arrogation of a power and an exercise in hypocrisy no longer acceptable. "[30] Gaylin puts these remarks in the context of saying that the techniques of modern science--genetic counseling and screening among them--should be judged by their possible benefits rather than their possible abuse.

Chapter 3

Abortion

The Cases

1   A woman is discovered to have developed cancer in the uterus during the last trimester of pregnancy (the last three months). A hysterectomy which will remove the cancerous growth before it spreads to other parts of the body will also, she is told, kill the fetus she is carrying. To protect her own life, the woman decides to have the operation.

2   A woman has mothered two children, and she and her husband decide they wish no more. She decides to practice contraception and has her physician fit her with an intra-uterine device (I.U.D.). After several years, she unexpectedly becomes pregnant due to a failure of the I.U.D. She and her husband decide to have the fetus aborted, rather than have their family planning interrupted.

3   An unmarried woman executive due for a promotion in a banking concern discovers that she is pregnant. The stigma she might have to endure by bearing an illegitimate child and the chance she might lose her position at her bank as a result lead to a decision to abort the fetus before anyone of her acquaintances, including the fetus's father, becomes aware of its existence.

The Issues

Abortion--the techniques of cutting or suctioning a fetus out of a mother's womb, or forcing a fatal premature delivery by using abortifacent drugs or solutions--is a form of birth control which can be used when contraception fails. In fact, according

to an exhaustive study of abortion, the ready availability of
abortion makes contraception users careless:

> In a change to a permissive system, restrictive countries with
> little or no tradition of contraception (Latin America, India) and
> which now have high criminal-abortion rates, probably would
> follow the pattern of current progressive countries before legal-
> ization (Eastern Europe, Japan) where traditional, frequently
> inefficient contraception was often supplemented by illegal
> abortion--that is, legal abortions would soar. [1]

Abortion also serves as a form of population control:

> Generally speaking, as countries become modernized, a declin-
> ing birthrate may be expected, accomplished mainly through
> abortion (legal or illegal) if effective contraceptives are not
> available or made acceptable by intensive education and promo-
> tion (U.S.S.R. before 1955). Abortion may decline as prosper-
> ity and use of contraception rises (Japan and Poland) but the
> birthrate will continue to decline (Japan and Poland). Thus, an
> increase in effective contraception may result in a decrease in
> abortions and a decrease in the birth rate. Finally, the most
> effective voluntary method of reducing a high birthrate would
> be a combination of a strong contraception program and permis-
> sive abortion laws. [2]

As a form of contraception and population control, abortion
raises the same ethical questions they do. Its own unique ethical questions arise from the fact that the life controlled is not
hypothetical, but the life of a living fetus that after ten weeks of
development looks very human indeed. The frequently reproduced pictures of the human-looking fetus sharpen and embitter
the arguments over its right to life and the rights of its mother
to live as she chooses in contemporary society.

Abortion is the one issue of medical ethics least likely to be
academic. Most people have debated its use; firsthand experience with abortion is more likely than with experimentation on
human subjects or with the allocation of an inadequate number
of kidney machines. With abortion, the problem of consent is
central. The process untherapeutically kills a form of human
life incapable of consenting to its own destruction in order to
serve the freedom of its mother to decide how to use her own
body and to run her own life. But a woman is freed from bond-

age to biology only by violating ancient religious and philosophical taboos against killing the inoffensive and defenseless.
The retort that the fetus is not human meets the strong objection that it is--a debate that inspired the impossible task of
defining just when human life begins, which leads to the even
more vexing task of defining what it is that is beginning. The
debate on abortion goes to the heart of what human beings think
they are and what they will or will not have science do to them.

A fair assessment of the enormous literature of abortion
would need to be as voluminous as Daniel Callahan's book on
abortion, already cited. The presentation in this chapter uses
an article Callahan developed out of the book to introduce two
typical arguments, one in defense of the life of the fetus, the
other the freedom of the mother. Both are then considered in
light of the Supreme Court's legal arbitration of the abortion
debate in its decision of 22 January 1973. Finally, we examine
a fresh approach to establishing a morality to fit the Court's
legal permissiveness, along with positive and negative reactions
to it. This would seem to get to the heart of the matter as
expeditiously as possible.

The Debate on Abortions

Daniel Callahan sees the debate on abortion pitting two
essentially valuable impulses against each other; rarely do the
proponents of one recognize the value of the other. The strength
of the pro-abortion movement lies in its efforts to correct two
elementary deficiencies. Woman have not had the freedom to
make their own choices in a matter critical to their development
as persons, and "the biological reality is that it is women who
become pregnant and bear children; nature gave them no choice.
Unless they are given a means to control the biological facts
and abortion is one very effective means--they will be dominated
by men. "[3] The strength of the anti-abortion movement lies in
its efforts to protect defenseless human life or potentially
human life. "It strives to resist the introduction into society
of forms of value judgements that would discriminate among
the worth of individual lives. "[4]

Respect for both arguments enables Callahan to detect the inadequacy of nine frequently heard arguments in the abortion debate:

1. Abortion is a religious issue or a philosophical issue, best left to the private conscience rather than to public legislation. "Not entirely," is his response. The practice or prohibition of abortion has consequences in the growth or decline of population. The fetus possibly has legal rights as a human being that the law should protect.

2. To remove restrictive abortion laws from the books passes no judgment on the substantive ethical issues--it merely allows individuals to make up their own minds. Again, he says, this argument ignores the social implications of the practice. The laws of the land do affect the consciences of those living in it; laws are needed to define the life and rights of the fetus.

3. Any liberalization of abortion laws or a repeal of such laws will lead in the long run to a disrespect for all human life. Callahan refers to the data (documented in his book) that shows this has not happened in countries such as Poland and Japan with almost twenty years of liberal abortion laws behind them. Furthermore it could be argued that the permissive abortion laws respect certain often neglected rights of the mother.

4. Scientific evidence, particularly modern genetics, has shown that human life begins at conception or at least at the time of implantation. On the contrary, the question when human life begins is philosophical, not scientific. Both the sperm and the egg are alive before conception, at which point begins a physiological development that strictly speaking doesn't cease until death. It is impossible to pinpoint one moment in the development of the fetus as being more essential than any other.

5. The fetus is nothing more than "tissue" or a "blueprint." "Tissue" is too vague a term. All forms of organic life can be considered as a complex of tissues. Blueprints exist apart from the edifices built according to their plan. The body of the fetus becomes an intrinsic part of the body of the child and the adult.

6. All abortions are selfish, ego-centered actions. To the contrary, often a mother will desire an abortion out of sense of obligation to living children so that they might enjoy a larger share of the family resources.

7. Abortions are "therapeutic" and abortion decisions are
"medical" decisions. Abortions are never therapeutic for the
fetus. And the mother usually is not seeking relief from a
physical or psychological defect when she asks for an abortion.
8. In a just society there would be no abortion problem since
the social and economic pressures that drive women to abortion
would not exist. In response Callahan points out that some wom-
en desire an abortion after a contraceptive failure; they use
the procedure to shape and plan their families according to
their own desires.
9. Abortion is exclusively a women's issue, to be decided by
women. The fetus is part of a woman's body; all too often the
male-dominated legislatures have been too insensitive to the
needs and feelings of women. Callahan points out that child-
bearing has consequences for everyone, not just women, then
adds: "Yet since I agree that abortion decisions should not
legally require the consent of husband and/or father--for I see
no way to include such a requirement in the law without opening
the way for further abuse of women--I am left with the (perhaps
pious) hope that there will be some recognition that problems of
justice towards the male are real (however new!) and that an
ethical resolution will be found. "[5]

Two Basic Positions

Robert F. Drinan, S. J., argues what Callahan considers the
strongest argument of the anti-abortion movement--all human
life, including its more helpless forms must be protected from
harm: "However convenient, convincing or compelling the arguments in favor of abortion may be, the fact remains that the
taking of a life, even though it is unborn, cuts out the heart of
the principle that no one's life, however unwanted and useless
it may be, may be terminated to promote the health or happiness of another human being. "[6]
At the beginning of his study, Drinan makes clear what to
him are non-issues. He is not arguing against abortion when
pregnancy imperils the mother's life, or results from rape or
incest. On the other hand, he understands that even arguments
in favor of abortion do not extend to viable fetuses and do not

intend abortion to become a substitute for birth control. At issue is the question of the abortion of a nonviable fetus upon demand of the mother for reasons of her own well-being. Drinan states that the tradition of common law forbids it, even when such a fetus is discovered to be "defective":

> I submit that it is illogical and intellectually dishonest for anyone to advocate as morally permissible the destruction of a defective non-viable fetus but to deny that this concession is not a fundamental compromise with what is one of the moral-legal absolutes of Anglo-American law--the principle that the life of an innocent human being may not be taken away simply because, in the judgement of society, nonlife for this particular individual would be better than life.[7]

He argues that the tradition of the law has protected society against brutalizing itself. Once it becomes an accepted practice to destroy fetuses, there is a danger that no line will be drawn against the killing of innocent but unwanted persons such as the sick, the mentally incompetent, the dying, or the crippled. Also, the tradition of the law has made a proper adjudication of the conflict between the rights to privacy and the rights to live. In the case of pregnancy, the right to live simply outweighs the right of a woman to the use of her own body as she wills.

Drinan responds to the frequently heard arguments that often an abortion is needed to protect the mental health of the mother by asking for studies to be made on the psychological effects which having an abortion has on the woman--to see whether the anguish caused by an abortion might approximate the anguish caused by not having one, and thus an assessment be possible that abortion simply replaces one kind of distress for another.

A psychiatrist, Richard A. Schwartz, cites such studies while arguing the strongest argument of the pro-abortion movement--women should have the freedom to make their own choice in a matter critical to their development as persons and to the development of society as a whole. He finds that studies made in this country and in Europe with several years' experience with permissive abortion laws shows that about 1 to 2 percent of the women studied experienced prolonged feelings of guilt or depression; most of them had been pressured against having abortions previously by friends, family, or clergy, or by their

own religious and moral beliefs. A large majority of women,
60 to 70 percent, experience no pangs of conscience at all. The
remainder do for a time, from a few weeks to a few months,
but then adjust, sometimes through the help of minimal counseling or therapy. By and large, he concludes, follow-up studies "strongly suggest that, contrary to folklore, serious psychiatric sequelae to abortion are relatively rare. Most women
tolerate the procedure quite well from the emotional standpoint. "[8]

Schwartz admits, however, that these studies are not completely reliable. They are few and far between, and often use
very different categories in their questionnaires. Few studies
have been made of the long-term psychological effects of an
abortion, perhaps after the woman who has long ago had an
abortion goes through menopause. Most of these studies, furthermore, were made of women having had legal abortions, whose
attitudes might be very different from the far greater majority
of women having had illegal abortions in many of the countries
surveyed. In addition, it is very likely that the experimenters
themselves were prejudiced. Psychiatrists tend to have liberal
attitudes towards abortion resulting from their contacts with the
middle-class women who want them. One could conclude that
Drinan's request is still to be adequately met.

But Schwartz takes a different tack. He surveys the studies
which suggest there is a great amount of psychiatric damage
done when abortions are not permitted or bungled badly by incompetent abortionists. A lack of access to abortion has been
shown to cause many forced marriages, for one thing, for which
the divorce rate is very high. Unwanted children are more
likely than loved children to require psychiatric care, to be
arrested, to go on welfare, to have drinking and drug problems.
"Psychiatrists generally agree that the single most important
cause of mental disorders is inadequate parental care during the
formative years. "[9]

What is particularly serious about these disorders, he says,
is that for the most part they cannot be adequately cured. Group
and individual psychotherapy and drugs work with relatively mild
disorders--neuroses, depressions, acute psychoses--not the
severe disorders such as chronic schizophrenia, alcoholism,
psychopathic personality, or chronic criminal behavior. The

realistic approach to the problem is preventive measures, and as it seems extremely difficult to intervene in family situations where unwanted children already exist, or to create substitutes for absent parental care, it would be best to diminish the numbers of unwanted children to begin with. One way to do this is to make contraception readily available. Often enough, however, contraception fails, or is not used by women who need it for reasons of poverty, ignorance, or lack of foresight:

> Unfortunately, analysis of the current state of birth control technology suggests there is little likelihood that we can significantly reduce the incidence of unwanted births in the foreseeable future without legalizing abortion. . . . Since abortion requires no foresight or self-discipline, legalization of abortion would make it possible for the most immature, emotionally unstable or mentally retarded woman to achieve total control over her reproduction . . . . The legalization of abortion is not a panacea, and will certainly not totally eliminate mental illness, but it is difficult to think of any single measure that would do more to reduce the incidence of serious psychiatric disorders.[10]

A Reflection on the Two Arguments

Strictly speaking, neither Drinan's nor Schwartz's argument explicitly mentions or defends the two basic positions Callahan described; rather, each assumes one tacitly. Drinan assumes the moral position that fetal life is worth more than a mother's perception of her well-being, while his argument is that in the question of abortion two laws or rights come into conflict, and that one outweighs the other by tradition and by logic. Schwartz assumes that the mother's right to privacy is at least equal to the fetus's right to live, while his argument is that social circumstances often tip the balance in favor of the former. Each tries as best he can to make a line of reasoning irrefutable in itself which can be plugged into support of their assumption. Yet the connection between their assumption and their reasoning remains rather arbitrary in both cases. One could argue against Drinan that despite the traditional bias against abortion in the law, there is no compelling reason not to change the law as times change. One could argue against Schwartz that the undesirable social consequences which arise from restricting abortion are

worth enduring to preserve the respect each individual life needs
for its society to endure.   If, on the other hand, either thinker
had made an absolute claim--abortion should not be permitted because all killing, except in self-defense or national defense, is
wrong or abortions should be permitted because a fetus isn't
human and lacks any human rights to weigh against the mother's--
there would be no possibility for discussion at all.   The abortion
debate goes on endlessly because the rival assumptions can't be
reconciled and all supportive or derivative arguments can be
refuted on their own merits, rather than on the assumptions which
underlie them.

This aside highlights the strategy the Supreme Court used to
arbitrate the abortion debate.   Depending on one's point of view,
their decision is a fascinating or maddening sidestep of either
assumption and most of the arguments which have been presented
in their defense.

The Supreme Court's Decision on Abortion

In its decision of 22 January 1973, the Supreme Court ruled
that a woman's right to privacy, protected without qualification
by the Fourteenth Amendment, outweighs the fetus's right to life
for the first six months of pregnancy.   A woman therefore may
request and receive an abortion in the first trimester of pregnancy
with a physician's approval.   No state can restrict the procedure
in any way.   She may also receive an abortion during the second
trimester subject only to the laws a state may pass to protect
the mother's health.   She may not have an abortion during the
period beginning with the last trimester of pregnancy, approximately at the time when the fetus has become viable, if the
state in which she resides passes laws forbidding it then.   This
the states may do to protect their interests in the individual.
But even during this time a woman may receive an abortion
if it is deemed necessary to save her life or health.   The Court
thus resolves the dilemma of conflicting rights by giving each
one its own time in which to reign: the woman's right for six
months, the fetus's for three.   (It could be argued that the fetus really doesn't have unalienable rights at all if a plea for a
woman's health could doom it even in the last three months.)

At first glance it might appear that the Court assumes that the moment of viability establishes the fetus as human with rights of its own. But throughout the decision the Court takes pains to keep its assumptions inaccessible and thus unassailable. The decision explicitly states that they do not wish to define the point at which life begins: "We need not resolve the difficult questions of when life begins. When those trained in the respective disciplines of medicine, philosophy, and theology are unable to arrive at any consensus, the judiciary at this point in the development of Man's knowledge is not in a position to speculate as to the answer. "[11]

All the Court does is to acknowledge that the rights of the mother and the fetus are distinct, that both are compelling, but the latter gains "substantiality" only as the fetus develops. "With respect to the states' important and legitimate interest in potential life, the <u>compelling</u> point is at viability.... State regulation protective of fetal life after viability has both logical and biological justifications"[12] (emphasis added). The Court is saying here that, strictly speaking, there are no hard reasons for seizing on this point in fetal development to serve as a turning point in a conflict of rights. The point must be established somewhere; this is a convenient place. Thus, by acknowledging no necessary connection between viability and the beginning of special fetal rights, the court cannot be attacked on strictly logical grounds for assigning the right at this point. It accepts the notion that both the mother and fetus have rights, but refrains from reasoning how they ought to be reconciled precisely. Their strategy is to have their judgment float free from any proofs from which it could be refuted.

To lend some support to their liberalization of the existing abortion laws, the Court finds persuasive (if not compelling) arguments of the kind Schwartz advanced. The times, society, and women have changed. So should the law:

The detriment that the State would impose upon the pregnant woman by denying this choice altogether is apparent. Specific and direct harm medically diagnosable even in early pregnancy may be involved. Maternity, or additional offspring, may force upon the woman a distressful life and future. Psychological harm may be imminent, mental and physical health may

be taxed by child care. There is also the distress, for all
concerned, associated with the unwanted child, and there is
the problem of bringing a child into a family already unable,
psychologically and otherwise, to care for it. In other cases,
as in this one, the additional difficulties and continuing stigma
of unwed motherhood may be involved. All these are factors
the woman and her responsible physician necessarily will
consider in consultation.[13]

In line with these reasons, the Court presents an elaborate
historical analysis of the trends in abortion laws--to serve as
a justification for their reversing the traditional laws against
it, and thereby to reject Drinan's concept that common law
should be taken as a norm. The survey begins with the ancient
laws about abortion and finds there a plurality of opinion. At
certain times and at certain places in the ancient world abortion
was permitted, and at others proscribed. Laws were relative
to the culture. The Court reasons that the problematic explicit prohibition of abortion in the Hippocratic Oath is likewise to be taken as culturally bound. The Court cites a scholar
Edelstein who points out that the oath was not uncontested
even in Hippocrates' day: "Only the Pythagorean school of
philosophers frowned upon the related act of suicide. Most
Greek thinkers on the other hand, commended abortion, at
least prior to viability. " [14]
The Court finds that in addition English common law initially
permitted abortion before quickening (sixteen to eighteen
weeks, or the time when the fetus could be felt moving inside
the mother). But the law remained ambiguous whether it
considered abortion of a fetus after quickening a crime. English statutory law vacillated in its restrictions on abortion
over time. The first American law in New York in 1828 held
it a misdemeanor to abort a fetus before quickening, second
degree manslaughter afterwards. But after this time began
a trend towards restricting abortion. "Gradually, in the
middle and late 19th century the quickening distinction disappeared from the statutory law of most states and the degree
of offense and the penalties were increased. By the end of
the 1950's a large majority of the States banned abortion, however and whenever performed, unless done to save or to pre-

serve the life of the mother. The exceptions, Alabama and the District of Columbia, permitted abortion to preserve the mother's health. "[15] The Court then goes on to view its own decision as legitimizing the most recent liberalizing trend away from only a relatively recent (and seemingly aberrant) century-old trend towards restriction. The Court's assumption--quite unacknowledged--seems to be that the present-day society needs abortion, so irrespective of any moral reasoning on either side or legal tradition, the law must be bent to the need.

Arguments Since the Court's Decision

Because the Court's decision is utilitarian rather than ethical, it is not surprising that ethical discussion about abortion has been heavy since it was handed down. Richard McCormick, S. J., a reviewer of the recent publications on the subject, wrote, "I have never seen so much writing in so concentrated a period of time on a single subject. "[16] From McCormick's review, it appears that for the most part writers have returned to previous ethical positions and sounded the drum for them more energetically.

One writer in particular has gained notice for a rather novel approach which can be seen as developing a moral thinking that might permit women to request the abortions now legally available to them with a sounder moral conscience. Judith Jarvis Thomson writes:

> I am arguing... that having a right to life does not guarantee having either a right to be given the use of or a right to be allowed continued use of another person's body--even if one needs it for life itself.... That no person is morally required to make large sacrifices to sustain the life of another who has no right to demand them, and this even where the sacrifices do not include life itself.... We are not morally required to be good Samaritans or anyway very good Samaritans to one another.[17]

She likens a woman being pregnant to a person who awakens one day to discover that during the night he has been kidnapped

and taken to a hospital where doctors have hooked up his kidneys
to the body of a famous violinist. The person is told that the
violinist's kidneys have failed and that he needs to be allowed
use of another's for a time to survive. He finds that the two
are strapped together back to back in the bed, with hoses con-
necting their kidneys. Thomson argues that because the process was begun without his permission, the person being tapped
is under no moral obligation to continue his being used in this
way. If he wished he could reach behind him and pull out the
violinist's hose without incurring any legal or moral fault. It
might perhaps be quite commendable and praiseworthy for him
not to pull the plug, of course. And it might be almost incum-
bent on him not to do so if told that the violinist only needed an
hour more of support to regain his health completely. But if
the violinist needed nine months or nine years of support, it
would be quite understandable if the unwilling donor ended the
violinist's dependence beforehand.

Thomson uses another analogy. She says that if all she
needed to recover from a fatal disease was to have Henry
Fonda lay his cool hand on her fevered brow, he would, strictly
speaking, be under no obligation to do so, as praiseworthy as
his doing so might be. If he were only on the other side of the
room when the request was made and he refused, the act would
be somewhat more surprising than if he were on a set two
thousand miles away, but in neither case would it be strictly
his duty to respond. Sacrifice always entails doing more than
one's strict duty. Viewed in these analogies, abortion is not
direct killing, but the removal of life support from an undesired
fetus.

Thomson goes on to reason that using such a model would be
moral only if the fetus has been truly unwanted all along; if its
conception was an accident due to a failure of birth control of
some kind. She rejects the possible objection that anyone who
enjoys sexual intercourse while using contraception should take
responsibility for any accidental pregnancy that might occur
because the risk was known beforehand. Thomson says that
would be tantamount to blaming a householder for a burglary of
his house just because the thief was able to force the lock.
Thompson also reasons that this model would prohibit abortion
after viability when the fetus no longer needed the mother's

support system to survive. Then it would be an independent
entity with rights to survival.

Thomson's arguments, it can be seen, develop a moral rational for what the Supreme Court permits legally. Following
her logic, a woman could in conscience and in the law abort a
fetus until the point when it becomes viable. Her arguments also
adroitly maneuver around the question of when human life begins
in the womb. The Court refused to define that point, and assumes
that determining that point precisely isn't required for the basis
of their decision. Thomson would grant the most conservative
assumption that life begins at conception (which is another way
of saying that the point when life begins cannot be determined
precisely), but then argues that a mother has no obligation to
sustain such a life unwillingly. Her example of a violinist is
especially appropriate because there is little doubt about accomplishment or worth to humanity; and as it is possible that
the kidnapped subject might be a male, the example gives a
reader of either sex a vicarious experience of involuntary responsibility for another life.

Three Responses to Thomson's Arguments

As can be seen from the date of publication, 1971, Ms.
Thomson herself did not intend her piece to be a response to the
Court's ruling in 1973. But more recently another ethician,
Sissela Bok, has drawn attention to Thomson's article, and has
shown how it can help define moral distinctions between abortions
and can justify on moral grounds some of the kinds of abortions
the Court allows. Bok builds on Thomson's arguments. She
points out that in using this model we would have to use methods
of abortion that actually did sever the support system rather
than kill the fetus outright: a method which prevents implantation of the fertilized egg; or, after the second trimester, a
hysterectomy, or "small Cesarean." Bok concentrates on
qualifying Thomson's position that the fetus can be considered
human and still be morally aborted, making unnecessary the
dangerous and always arbitrary distinction between who is human
and what is not. A good approach, Bok reasons, would be to
consider why we prohibit the murder of living human beings, in

order to see if any of these reasons apply to the fetus. She
lists four:

    1. Killing is viewed as the greatest of all dangers for the victim.
--The knowledge that there is a threat to life causes intense anguish and apprehension.
--The actual taking of life can cause great suffering.
--The continued experience of life, once begun, is considered so
valuable, so unique, so absorbing, that no one who has this experience should be unjustly deprived of it. And depriving someone of this experience means that all else of value to him will be
lost.
    2. Killing is brutalizing and criminalizing for the killer. It is
a threat to others, and destructive to the person engaged therein.
    3. Killing often causes the family of the victim and others to
experience grief and loss. They may have been tied to the dead
person by affection or economic dependence; they may have
given of themselves in the relationship, so that its severance
causes deep suffering.
    4. All of society, as a result, has a stake in the protection of
life. Permitting killing to take place sets patterns for victims,
killers, and survivors that are threatening and ultimately harmful to all.[18]

Bok argues that in light of these reasons, the need to protect
lives from abortion in the very early stages of cell formation
are minimal. All that one denies the fetus is potential. After
quickening (at the end of the first trimester), however, more
of the reasons against killing begin to come into play. And
after viability (approximately at the end of the second trimester),
almost all do; in fact, killing the viable fetus can be considered
tantamount to infanticide. Her conclusions also fit within the
Court's guidelines restricting somewhat the moral grounds for
abortion in the second and third trimester:

Before quickening, the reasons to protect life are, as has been
shown, negligible, perhaps absent altogether. During this
period, therefore, abortion could be permitted upon request.
Alternatively, the end of the first trimester could be employed
as such a limit, as is the case in a number of countries.
    Between quickening and viability, when the operation is a
more difficult one medically and more traumatic for parents
and medical personnel, it would not seem unreasonable to

hold that special reasons justifying the abortion should be
required in order to counterbalance this resistance; reasons
not known earlier, such as the severe malformation of the fetus.
After viability, finally, all abortions save the rare ones required to save the life of the mother, should be prohibited,
because the reasons to protect life many not be thought to be
partially present; even though the viable fetus cannot fear death
or suffer consciously therefrom, the effects on those partici-
pating in the event, and thus on society indirectly, could be
serious. This is especially so because of the need, mentioned
above, for a protection against infanticide. In the unlikely
event, however, that the mother should first come to wish to
be separated from the fetus at such a late stage, the procedure
ought to be delayed until it can be one of premature birth, not
one of harming the fetus in an abortive process.[19]

Thomson's article has been attacked on grounds that her
distinction between non-sustaining life and direct killing is
not valid in the case of a fetus who only knows life at this point
as sustained life. Its only life is such a qualified life, and it
has as much a right to its own kind of life as adults do to theirs.
Baruch Brody argues that furthermore one has a duty to save
or to preserve a dependent life when "there is so little to
lose." He doesn't think that the woman's right to privacy
can be considered on the same plane as a right to life.[20]
John Finnis argues that the child has a right to life from
another source than the mother's granting it either implicity
or explicitly: "...What Thomson...fails to attend to adequately
is the claim (one of the claims implicit, I think, in the papal
and conservative rhetoric of rights) that the mother's duty not
to abort herself is not an incident of any special responsibility
which she assumed or undertook for the child, but is a straight-
forward incident of an ordinary duty everyone owes his neighbor."[21] His use of the word "neighbor" indicates that for
Finnis, the fetus is the mother's equal in its right to life. No
nicety of language, he goes on to say, can make the "removing
of life support" anything less than killing.

Chapter 4

Behavior Control–
Psychotropic Drugs,
Behavior Modification,
and Psychosurgery

The Cases

1   A radical political activist is arrested for causing a dis-
turbance at a political rally. She resists arrest and fights
with the jailer. After being placed in a cell, she calms down
and goes to sleep. When she is arraigned the next day, she at
first appears very docile, then suddenly flies into a rage and
attempts to attack the judge, accusing him of being an "enemy
of the people." As she appears to have no family or financial
means, the judge commits her to a state hospital for observation, but after several days she begins to accuse the staff
and the inmates of plotting against her because of her radical
political views. She starts several fights. A physician assigned to the case suggests to the patient and her court-appointed
lawyer that she be sedated with the antipsychotic drug Taractin
while under observation. The lawyer agrees, but the patient
flies into a rage when asked by the doctor for her consent. She
accuses him of trying to poison her. She is asked several days
later with the same reaction. In the interim, she has had
several more fights with the attendants. Finally, after consulting with the hospital staff, the doctor orders her to be
forcibly sedated. Afterwards she remains calm for several
days and even becomes eager to please. When the drug's
dramatic effect is pointed out to her, she herself requests that
the therapy be continued.

2   An American Indian reservation in the Northwest is suffering from psychic and financial depression. For 150 years they
have refused to have any interactions with white Americans out
of a deep and lasting anger at being displaced from their tribal
lands on the plains. Until recently, they have survived well

enough by subsistence farming, hunting and fishing, and by
trade with neighboring tribes. They still practice their ances-
tral religions and so are considered somewhat old fashioned by
their neighboring tribes, who aren't very concerned with their
current plight. Severe rainstorms have destroyed the tribe's
crops for several years. Their numbers have dwindled as
young members of the tribe have left the reservation. The
tribe, the elders say sadly, is returning to the earth.

Some of the younger members of the tribe who do not wish to
leave the reservation secretly petition the Bureau of Indian
Affairs for help. An agent who is himself a full-blooded Indian
is sent. He can speak the tribe's language and after several
days of presenting his credentials he wins the elders' respect.
After assessing the tribe's situation, he suggests that they sell
some land to another reservation to raise capital. With it they
can set up a small electronics plant that will do commission work
for plants on other reservations that assemble products for a
national market. At first the elders are reluctant. The agent
describes the plan in more detail. The elders are to be appointed
overseers of the project, to be guided initially by the agent himself who has a degree in psychology and business administration.
The younger members of the tribe will be given responsibility
according to their age at first, then, after on-the-job training
(organized by Indians from other reservations), according to
their expertise. At any time after the project begins, the elders
can decide to abandon it.

After much argument the elders finally agree to try the project. The elders are kept in titular posts while the agent actually
runs the business, and sees to the steady advancement in expertise and salary of the more gifted younger members of the tribe.
The company begins to bring substantial profits to the tribe's
treasury. It buys back the land it originally sold, and under
guidance from the agent begins to purchase home building mat-
erials, at first using other Indians as middlemen and then, to
cut down on costs, directly from nationally franchised cut-rate
lumber companies. Their old animosity toward the white man
is almost forgotten. Many members of the tribe who had moved
away begin to move back. A representative from General
Electric asks the tribal elders if his company can locate a small

factory on the reservation to take advantage of the good labor market and lack of a need to pay property taxes. With the approval of the agent, the elders readily agree, immensely satisfied with the new vitality of their community.

3   A man is arrested repeatedly for making sexually sugges-tive remarks to young children and exposing himself. Finally he serves a five-year sentence in an institute for the criminally insane. After seeming to rehabilitate himself through group therapy sessions and by learning a manual trade, he is paroled with the understanding that he will be immediately incarcerated if he is found to be sexually deviant again. Once outside he finds it hard to relate to other adults at his job and fears that his old patterns of behavior might repeat themselves. While institutionalized he had heard of a psychosurgical operation called hypothalamectomy which makes a lesion in the hypothal-amic section of the brain and has been demonstrated to blunt sexual urges. He locates a surgeon willing to perform the operation on him, provided the parole board agrees to it. They refuse. Their argument is that their duty is to monitor the normal behavior of a paroled convicted criminal, not to allow him to experiment with changing his state of mind.

The Issues

Recently developed behavior-control technology has made spectacular advances in treating mental disabilities, from MBD-- minimal brain dysfunction, most often called hyperactivity syndrome--to the involuntary homicidal rages of certain types of epileptics. In 1937 it was discovered that doses of ampheta-mines which can excite adults seem paradoxically to calm hyperkinetic (hyperactive) children. These children often run around like human dynamos, act up in classrooms, and find it difficult to pay attention to anything for an extended period of time. The drug seems to "stimulate" greater restraint which can have a domino effect on the child's behavior. As the child becomes more attentive, he wins more praise for his work and finds it easier to get along with other children. Self-esteem increases. When the drug was used with the more difficult children in an institution for delinquent children, all the children became more manageable. [1]

Since World War II, the development and administration of other psychotropic drugs, those which influence the mind and alter behavior, mood, and mental functioning, such as anti-psychotics (tranquilizers) antidepressants (amphetamines), and antianxiety drugs (Librium, Valium, and so forth), have had a dramatic impact on the treatment of mental diseases in adults. The drugs seem to balance chemical instability in the brain, making it possible for a patient to lead a more normal life in the face of otherwise unbearable stress. More patients can be treated at home, where there is more free space and less violence than in hospitals. The stigma attached to mental illness has lessened. Patients can adjust to their normal life situations more easily.[2]

Since the 1940s and mostly under the influence of B. F. Skinner, a Harvard psychologist and behaviorist, techniques of behavior modification have become very sophisticated. Pavlov's earlier experiments in conditioning a dog to respond to artificial stimulus associated with a natural stimulus (salivating to the sound of a bell that was rung many times while meat was being presented) have led to the development of operant conditioning--changing the reinforcements of a behavior in order to change the behavior. A smug inmate of a mental institution who does no work and yet is fed anyway is told that from now on only work will earn food. Doing no work (the undesired behavior) now leads to no food (a new negative reinforcement); working (the desired behavior) leads to food (a new positive reinforcement). An American psychiatrist, Lloyd H. Cotter, described the effect operant conditioning had on a Vietnamese mental hospital during the war. When he arrived in 1966, he found the hospital with very poor morale, with diminishing stores of food and drugs. He decided to attack the problems of lassitude and lack of food simultaneously. Patients were told they had to work if they ever hoped to be discharged. A small number volunteered. Those who refused were immediately given unmodified electroconvulsive treatments on a regular basis. After some weeks, many were helped by the treatment; others improved greatly when, through dislike of the treatment, they joined the work force.

Later Cotter changed his tactics by adding another reinforcement. He told the patients still not working that if they didn't do some work, they wouldn't be fed. After three days, almost all of the patients were working. He comments:

> The argument that subjecting these patients to electro-
> convulsive treatments or withholding food might be considered
> cruel was countered by the comparison to a child with pneu-
> monia receiving antiobiotic injections. The injections hurt and
> even involve some slight risk to the patient, but the damage
> without their use is potentially much greater. Inflicting a little
> discomfort to provide motivation to move patients out of their
> zombie-like states of inactivity, apathy, and withdrawal was,
> in our opinion, well justified.
>
> As time passed it became evident that even the patients felt
> this way. As I made my way among large groups of these newly
> working patients, who were clearing fields with their hands
> and with hoes in order to plant crops to help alleviate the food
> shortage, I was not struck or threatened. Instead I was greeted
> with smiles and comments which indicated that they were more
> satisfied with themselves in their more productive and useful
> roles and grateful to us for having pushed them into it. [3]

Similar techniques have been used to toilet train seriously disturbed children, and to teach them to interrelate with other
people and even to speak and read.[4]

In the early 1950s, James Olds inspired an enormous amount
of research into techniques for exploring and changing the brain
when he implanted an electrode into the brain of a rat and found
he could alter its behavior and mood by switching the current on
and off. The therapeutic psychosurgery which has developed--
lobotomy, electric stimulation of the brain (ESB), and other
techniques that cut or coagulate with electrical current parts of
the brain--has enabled doctors to blunt tension and anxiety, and
to control violence in patients who don't respond to either drugs
or psychological conditioning. In the process the surgeons have
attracted sharp ethical questioning by their presumption to cure
sickness by changing the patient permanently--not into a healthy
person which not even conventional medicine can presume to
do--but into a different person. Even before the electrical
probe or knife touches the target area of the operation, it has
cut through a delicate structure of neurological relays that eons
of human evolution and perhaps decades of personal experience
have shaped. Psychosurgery, probably more than any other

branch of medicine, is developing a formative rather than curative science.

In 1970, two neurosurgeons, Vernon H. Mark and Frank R. Ervin, reported the case of a patient, Thomas, an epileptic with a history of seizures and episodes of uncontrollable, murderous rages. He would suddenly and without provocation try to harm members of his family. It was determined that certain types of epileptic electrical activity triggered the rages even at times when there was no overt indication that a seizure was taking place or imminent. He did not respond to treatment with psychotropic drugs.

The surgeons inserted electrodes into Thomas's brain which they could use to stimulate different parts of his brain in order to discover which part, when stimulated, brought on the symptoms of one of his rages. For three months they kept him free of rages through the electrical stimulation of his relaxation mood whenever he appeared about to fall into his mood of anger. After this period of observation they determined that, having located the diseased part of the brain with certitude, it was time to operate to neutralize it, to make the patient's therapy permanent. After stimulating him to relax, they asked his consent. He agreed and was happy with his decision until the effects of his stimulation faded, at which point he "turned wild and unmanageable," absolutely refusing any further therapy. Only after several weeks of patient explanation were the doctors able to convince Thomas to have the lesion of his brain made. "Four years have passed since the operation, during which time Thomas has not had a single episode of rage." [5]

Lobotomy, a lesion along the midline base of the frontal lobe, treats more generalized unmanageability. At first, in the 1950s, it was widely used in this country to sedate chronically ill patients in mental institutions. Some fifty thousand operations were performed. More recently it has been used to treat hyperactive children and neurotics. An Indian, Dr. Balasubraminian, reporting his results with 115 patients (three of them under the age of five, thirty-six under eleven), indicates why it was and is again becoming popular: "The improvement that occurs has been remarkable. In one case a patient had been assaulting his colleagues and the ward doctors; after the operation he became

a helpful addition to the ward staff and looked after other
patients. " [6]

A German experimenter, F. D. Roeder, recently made
lesions in the hypothalamic region to cure a patient of sexually
deviant behavior. In his report he writes, "Potency was
weakened, but preserved.... The aberrant sexuality of this
patient was considerably suppressed, without serious side-
effects. The important feature was the patient's incapacity of
indulging in erotic fancies and stimulating visions. " [7]

All three forms of behavior control work to shape the "will"
of a person, a philosophic term for the control a person exer-
cises over his or her behavior. It is easy to see how it could
be used for the good of a patient like Thomas--who might be
better able to control embarrassing, inefficient, or self-
destructive impulses--and for the good of his family and society
at large. Restrained personalities are easier for everyone to
live with. At the same time, it is easy to see how behavior control could be used for ill, especially if the physician deciding
what inadequate self-control is and what adequate medical
controls are doesn't share the views of either the patient or
other members of the society. The American doctor, Cotter,
for example, doesn't consider it important to determine
whether his Vietnamese inmates' attitudes towards work might
be shaped by their very different culture or their experiences
in the war. According to his report, his decision to change
their habitual behavior seemed to be even to them the right one.
The problem is perhaps more acute when patients are unruly
rather than too passive. How well could a physician draw the
line between erratic social behavior and radical social action
between a patient who disrupts the order of a hospital because
he is sick and tired of an injustice he perceives there, or
another who disrupts it because he is just sick?

The Ethics of Drugging

Robert Veatch describes five different categories of "ethics"
which people use in dispensing and consuming drugs. [8] His
categories work for distinguishing attitudes governing the use
of other behavior control technologies as well. So expanded,

they can help plot a way through the ethical arguments over behavior control reviewed in this chapter.

Patients and doctors who share the "Wisdom of Nature Ethic" would be loath, Veatch says, "to poison" the body with any substance, especially those which control such fundamentally human complexities as behavior, mood, or experience. The body and mind should endure what comes and cure itself.

The other drug ethics are more interventionist. Believers in the "Protestant Drug Ethic" will do what is necessary to get people back to work. Coffee is an approved drug; marijuana is not. Doses of tranquilizers or amphetamines turned to making the patient more stable and efficient are acceptable. Veach cites an advertisement for Ritalin (methylphenidate) run in medical magazines which promises to control a hyperkinetic child's "purposeless activity."[9] Believers in the "Neo-Protestant Drug Ethic," on the other hand, will help themselves or others to reach enlightenment or salvation with certain carefully selected chemicals, such as LSD, peyote, and other hallucinogens. It might seem very different from the more traditional "Protestant Ethic," Veatch says, since the goal is pleasure, not work. But each is a search for salvation using man-made means, and the second can be considered the offspring of the first (just as middle-class kids using LSD are often the offspring of parents using tranquilizers).

Believers in the "Protean Drug Ethic" will sample, mix, and balance many experiences with no attempt to integrate them into a common core of meaning. "For the drug user who is a protean man, the medicine chest will be a full one." But such a man is not very likely to be a physician. A physician and a growing number of middle-aged and middle-class people are more likely to hold to the "Therapeutic Drug Ethic," which retains the pluralism of the "Protean Drug Ethic" but integrates drug use with social goals. The highest is "fitting in"; the "achievement of a state of harmony, 'adjustment,' or equilibrium.... The goal is to diminish the perceptual dissonance by decreasing the perception."[10] Antianxiety and antidepressant agents are esteemed. An ad for Milparth (meprobamate and tridihexethyl chloride) promises "to keep the constant complainer from becoming an office fixture."[11] Veatch concludes "These five value-sets or world views... constitute the major

framework for decisions to use chemical agents to control
human behavior, mood, or experience. ... Others might be
added and no one value-set will be the total basis for drug
taking and drug-prescribing decisions. Some combination of
these or some alternative evaluative orientation must be the
basis of all such decision. " 12

Veatch's categories underscore the political nature of the
debate over psychotropic drugs (and other forms of behavior
control as well, using different means for comparable ends).
Control is power, even if over a single patient, and even if the
controller seeks only to control himself. The argument is over
who controls whom how. He reasons further that certain guidelines for drugging could follow from his analysis. A doctor
should prescribe mind-altering drugs that fit into his patient's
drug ethic, not solely his own; and by the same token, both
physician and layman should abide by the drug regulations that
represent the Weltanschauung of the culture they live in. But
he hopes that "a high value in individual freedom including the
right to control one's own body chemistry might be an important part of that Weltanschauung. " 13

The "Protestant Drug Ethic"

Lester Grinspoon and Susan Singer in an article on the
treatment of hyperactive children place the persons they see as
indiscriminate dispensers of amphetamines to hyperactive children in the "Protestant Ethic" camp and condemn both the
attitude and the sloppy research which serves it. They cite a
report of parents complaining that they have been pressured by
school boards to permit their children to be drugged:

> The Christian Science Monitor reported a southern California
> mother as saying, "We've been harassed and pressured by the
> school for four years now to put our nine-year-old on medica-
> tion--for hyperactivity--and we've refused for four years. Two
> family doctors have backed up our decision. " A Colorado
> mother told how she had reluctantly "caved in to the combined
> requests of the school nurse, the school psychologist, princi-
> pal, and teachers" that she put her six-year-old son on medi-
> cation to treat his "learning disability. " Another California
> mother complained that the school would not accept a "no" from

a family physician. "Most every parent who has an overactive child in the school is told to go see the same pediatrician," she reported, "because that doctor knows what the school wants." Even in cases where parents have not resisted and perhaps have even supported teachers' pressures to place their children on stimulants, a question still arises about whether educators should have any authority in making such recommendations. [14]

Behind such pressure, Grinspoon and Singer suspect one could find the overweening desire of teachers and principals for orderly classrooms--a desire that might cause a blurring of the distinction between hyperactivity and healthy aggressiveness. Their suspicion is strengthened for them when they discover in their literature research that the immediate effects have been too dramatic and gratifying to encourage careful scrutiny of the precise cause of the unwanted behavior:

> The behavior taken as a sign of hyperkinesis is real enough.
> Restless, angry, disturbed, and inattentive students constitute
> a major problem for many parents and teachers. It also may
> be true that some elementary school children exhibit this kind
> of behavior because of organic brain damage or neurohormonal
> insufficiencies. But it is impossible to believe that the 200,000
> or more school children who are now being routinely adminis-
> tered stimulants are all suffering from organic brain damage
> or deficiencies in crucial CNS chemicals. In other words,
> there is no justification for the increasingly popular leap from
> the observation of disruptive or inattentive behavior to the sup-
> position that this is the result of a specific disorder of the
> central nervous system. Nor does the observation that amphet-
> amines sometimes reduce disruptiveness and increase attention
> provide any grounds for supposing that even these are true
> cases of organically-based hyperkinesis. As we have seen,
> amphetamines can affect behavior and learning problems of
> psychogenic and environmental etiology in much the same way
> as they affect problems presumed to have an organic basis. [15]

Grinspoon and Singer have another complaint echoed by Peter Breggin in his equally comprehensive review of the prac- tice of psychosurgery. It is that the dramatic effects of these technologies have tended to make them resistent to closely controlled studies attesting their long-term effects. Our society in a sense is carrying out serious experiments with human subjects that aren't even advancing science very efficiently.

Political Implications

Other writers fear that political intolerance for deviant behavior of all kinds could also work conveniently to blur the distinction between uncontrollable energy and aggressive rebelliousness. Doctors pursuing either the "Neo-Protestant" or the "Therapeutic" ethic could order them into the service of ideology. Seymour L. Halleck writes, "What would be the political consequences of 'curing' the aggressiveness of a Malcolm X or an Eldridge Cleaver?"[16] Thomas Szasz writes: "The expression 'mental illness' is a metaphor that we have come to mistake for a fact. We call people physically ill when their body-functioning violates certain anatomical and physiological norms; similarly, we call people mentally ill when their personal conduct violates certain ethical, political, and social norms. This explains why many historical figures, from Jesus to Castro, and from Job to Hitler, have been diagnosed as suffering from this or that psychiatric malady."[17] What if the controls for the electrodes implanted in Thomas's brain fell into the hands of a leader who could, by pushing the buttons for pain or pleasure make of Thomas a willing slave or of a nation of Thomases an empire?

The Problem of Consent

The most effective check against such outlandish schemes would be the consent process, of course, just as it is the most effective check against all possible abuses of medical technology. But the case of Thomas serves to suggest how much more problematic consent is when a doctor is dealing with a patient whose very malady the doctor is trying to cure could be clouding the patient's judgment. Thomas consented when he had been stimulated to relax, when he was not in his natural mind, so to speak. But when the stimulation faded and he flew into a rage at the suggestion that his brain be cut into, he could be said to be out of his right mind and equally unable to make a valid consent. On top of this, the operation was intended quite literally to change his mind and to change Thomas into a different kind of person than his abnormal brain had made him. At the time when Thomas withdrew his consent,

he didn't seem to think the change was worth it. Clearly there
was no firm ground in his case in which to securely anchor the
consent process.

Cognizant of this danger, Robert Neville reasons that the
new powers of behavior-control technology give their wielders
a greater responsibility than medical practitioners have had before. No one has the access inside a human personality that
they do: "Now we have scientific technologies for manipulating
people inside the perimeters of their conscious defenses. Psychosurgery, drugs, behavior modification, and other forms of
psychotherapy manipulate people in the connections lying in
between their symbolic interpretation of the world and their
consciously intended responses. This is like saying that within
the processes of the mind we have found a body on which we can
operate. " [18]

The "uncontrollable" patient is particularly vulnerable to a
physician practicing what Veatch called the "Therapeutic Ethic. "
Neville says that mental health medicine has often adopted the
same standards of physical medicine: the goal of the latter is to
make a person's parts work as a harmoniously integrated system; the goal of the former can become making a person a part
of a harmoniously integrated society.

A better standard for behavior control, he thinks, would be
the rehabilitation of the patient's own unique integrity; the
maximizing of an individual's various capacities of response
in some compatible harmony with each other. A troubled person
should be helped again to take advantage of a variable environment. A troubled sax player should be helped to play the blues
better, a lonely woman to cope with her loneliness, a social
critic to criticize society better. Along with this behavior,
medicine should recognize the "right of the person in his
integrity to refuse the demands and services of the public environment except in the cases where his refusal jeopardizes
the environment itself or the integrity of the others in it" [19]
(emphasis added). Individuals could choose to put other things
above someone else's definition of what good mental health
means. Prisoners would be permitted to be or not to be re-
habilitated into society at their own pace, not forced to speed
the process up with the use or threat of medicine.

Neville's exception, of course, lets back in almost as much
of dilemma as his insistence on respect for the integrity of
an individual removes. Who is to make a decision when a
patient's refusal to be medicated becomes a case which en-
dangers the integrity of others? In the absence of a patient's
heroic hold on his own integrity, we need an almost heroic
discretion of a doctor assessing how much and how little to do
about an individual's disturbing behavior. Right-to-treatment
laws often intensify the dilemma. Many states require that
patients committed to mental institutions be treated for the
cause of their commitment; they cannot be kept in mere custodial care. What of a patient's right to refuse treatment in such
a case--especially if he or she is prone to homicidal rages that
could threaten other inmates?

Seymour Halleck develops some guidelines for the physicians
attending these kinds of cases:

> I do not feel there is ever ethical justification for deceiving the
> patient. All patients, even the most disturbed, should be in-
> formed of what will be done to them, why it will be done, and
> what effects the treatment is likely to have. If after having
> such information, the patient still does not consent to treat-
> ment, coercive treatment is justified only if the following sets
> of conditions are met:
>
> First, the patient must be judged to be dangerous to himself
> or others. In the case of civilly committed patients, this judge-
> ment has often been made in the process of commitment.
>
> Second, those who are providing treatment must believe
> there is a reasonable probability that treatment will be of
> benefit to the patient as well as to those around him.
>
> Third, the patient must be judged to be incompetent to
> evaluate the necessity for treatment. . . .
>
> The decision to impose treatment upon a non-consenting
> patient requires extraordinarily complex medical and ethical
> judgements. I do not believe that such decisions should be made
> by a single doctor except in emergencies. For that matter,
> such decisions should be made by groups of doctors working
> in the same institutional setting without the benefit of some
> outside monitoring and feedback. [20]

He goes on to propose that a monitoring board include the patient's physician, a psychiatrist, and an attorney. Such a

process would be expensive, he admits, but "it would serve as
a message to society that even the most disturbed individuals
are not to be subjected to behavior control without careful
consideration."[21]

Vernon H. Mark (who along with Frank R. Ervin wrote <u>Violence
and the Brain</u>) develops in an article co-authored by Robert
Neville the guidelines he would use as a physician to regulate
the practice of psychosurgery. The authors think as Halleck
does that "a committee of some sort, composed of physicians,
lawyers, ethicists, and perhaps patient advocates" should monitor the process. But they would even limit the kinds of surgery
that should even be allowed to come up for question: "Medical
procedures as drastic as neurosurgery should be used only
when behavior is abnormal and bad primarily because of an
abnormality in the brain. Abnormal violent behavior <u>not</u> associated with brain disease should be dealt with politically and
socially and not medically."[22] They would further restrict its
use to correction of brain damage only when it caused unwarranted and unprovoked acts that directly attempt to or
actually do injure or destroy another person or thing. "This
does not include violence consistently organized for a political
motive."[23] In short, they restrict the use of psychosurgery to
patients suffering from uncontrolled, violent behavior related
to epilepsy.

They go on to say that they would deny its use to any other
kind of patient, even if the individual begged for it--because
he or she might be influenced by pressure from friends or
society to become more normal. They would also deny it to the
prisoner because "it is particularly impossible to divorce the
moral connotations of the criminal status from evaluation for
therapeutic purposes of the person's pathological characteristics.
Therefore, the integrity of the therapeutic motive is systematically in jeopardy of gross distortion by motives of punishment
or custodial docility."[24]

There are several problems that arise when one tries to use
this guideline, however. <u>All</u> behavior, normal and abnormal,
has organic roots in the chemistry and electrical circuitry of
the brain. A physician could turn this restriction into a license
to cut away at will. In fact, if the mental illness comes to be

considered another "physical" deformity, it might even become
mandatory to operate on the "abnormal" brain as it is now on a
failing heart. Finally, cutting into a brain to get at some
diseased material or to insert wires means cutting through
healthy brain tissue as well, and destroying it in the process.
Breggin writes: "Since the brain is such a delicately balanced
instrument with unimaginable inter-relations, senseless mutilation of one part or another can disrupt the harmony still further, resulting in a general subduing of the organism and a general malfunction of his adaptational process."25
    A doctor's respect for a patient's integrity and, however
much it is possible to create, a covenant of consent between
doctor and patient, appear to be the only safeguards in behavior
control technology. The biological model can be manipulated;
monitoring boards could be loaded; legal guidelines could be
justified by reference to the need for institutional safety if a
physician in control of uncontrollable patients wanted to use
his or her power solely to serve a personal ethic. Neville
and Halleck fear that too often behavior modifiers will assume
"Therapeutic" or "Protestant" ethics and impose them on
helpless patients who might not share them. Judging from
the cases Grinspoon, Singer, Breggin, Mark and Ervin, and
Roeder and Cotter document, the fear is salutary.

Utopian Schemes of Control

    Two other thinkers have very different views of consent.
They envision a day when behavior modification might render
consent superfluous. Humans could be made perfectly content
with the world they live in, freed from chance and choice.
José M. R. Delgado, a professor of physiology and a developer
of many techniques of psychosurgery, has come to believe that
because all human experience resides in the brain, the best
way to make humans happier and healthy is to alter the brain
directly, treating it as a machine that can be tuned up, bypass-
ing the more complicated tasks of changing the environment
which shapes it. In speaking of the alleviation of fear, he moves
easily from discussing how electric stimulation of the brain
can help cure the sick to how it might change a whole society.
    Fear, he says, is only a certain pattern of electrical and
chemical activity in the brain that individuals learn to associate

with certain cultural experiences. Having learned now how to
stimulate fear artificially in a patient hooked up to a machine
that sends out electrical impulses, we stand ready to make an
exhaustive "exploration of the neuronal mechanisms of anxiety. "[26] We should be able eventually to map the movements
of fear through the thalamus, amygdala, and determine how
they signal the release of chemicals into the glands and muscles. We would gain for the first time an objective view of
what has always seemed a mysterious human activity; this view
would provide the basis for designing new drugs and psychiatric
treatments for many suffering patients. It might even lead to
programs for ameliorating anxiety in our civilization. We
would cut it off from its roots in the brain.

In other places, his enthusiasm for a man-made humanity
is even more explicit. He writes in the preface to The Physical
Control of the Mind: Toward a Psycho-civilized Society: "The
thesis of this book is that we now possess the necessary technology for the experimental investigation of mental activities,
and that we have reached a critical turning point in the evolution of man at which the mind can be used to influence its own
structure, functions, and purpose, thereby ensuring both the
preservation and advance of civilization. "[27] One of the techniques he describes in the book is the remote control of other
human beings by means of electrodes planted in the brain and
manipulated by an observer, a procedure that has already been
developed to work with primates and humans. Patients have been
stimulated to express affection and sexual interest in the thera-
pist. According to Delgado, this has enormous promise for
making psychotherapy more efficient. "Psychoanalysis requires
a long time and a person can easily withdraw his cooperation and
refuse to express intimate thoughts. "[28] Not so, it seems, if the
patient is on the machine. In another place he describes how
a patient was made to reveal deep-rooted anxieties about his
sexual identity that he was otherwise able to keep to himself.[29]

He labels opponents of his vision as romanticists, overly
fond of outdated concepts of "freedom, " "individuality, " and
"spontaneity" that simply stand in the way of permitting science
to help humans escape their brute past. In a recent discussion
held at Hastings Center, he stated: "I'm not satisfied with the

way in which our present civilization is behaving. I do not
believe that we must be slaves of natural chance. Up to now
man has been structured in a natural way by nature. And the
results are that we are full of flaws. We should improve the
society in which we live. ... The inviolability of the brain is only
a social construct, like nudity. "[30]

Peter Breggin responds to Delgado's book: "Delgado is the
theoretician of the lobotomist, the great apologist for Technological Totalitarianism, complete with an outright attack on
'liberal' politics, meaning not the liberalism of the left, but
principles of personal autonomy, independence and freedom, man's
'unalienable right' as annunciated in the Declaration of Independence. "[31] Peter London responded to Delgado's remarks in the
discussion by pointing out Delgado's principal assumption that it
would be preferable consciously to program man than to let man
continue to develop randomly, then adds: "The randomness of
that system may not be unfortunate. And possibly the randomness
and our lack of control over this system of informational input
into the nature of man, this post genetic rather than genetic random input, may also not be unfortunate. "[32]

B. F. Skinner's visions for a behavior-controlled society are
even grander and have excited even more energetic criticism.
We consider both in some detail. Arguments over Skinner's
theory dispute how much respect is due unique, unexpected, or
"random" human behavior. If that behavior is thought to be
genuinely unpredictable, respect for it often goes along with a
willingness to endure the antics of both sinners and saints, thieves
and artists, freaks and straights. There is a belief that you
can't have one kind of freedom without the other; to endure one
is to permit the other. But if that behavior is thought to be
merely the result of unusual conditions which, if known, would make
the behavior utterly predictable (if, in short, a genuine free will
is thought not to exist at all), then one might be more likely to go
along with Skinner's idea of conditioning all behavior benevolently,
homogenizing saints and sinners into good, respectable citizens.
The social dimension of all forms of behavior control lies directly
on the surface of this issue; what is said about Skinner's theory
can flow back over all that is said about all its other forms, including Delgado's utopian psychosurgery.

The basis of Skinner's theory is his analysis of behavior into three component parts: Stimulus, which causes Behavior as its reaction, which is followed by Reinforcement (any change, result, or reward stemming from the behavior).   Learning for Skinner is a process of feedback where Reinforcement continually sharpens and refines the Stimulus.   The Reinforcement of feeling safer improves the Behavior of running up a tree in a young squirrel who fears a sudden noise (Stimulus).   The Reinforcement of feeling satisfied improves the Behavior of asking for milk in a child who is thirsty (Stimulus).   In each example, both the subject and the environment "change"; the squirrel is now in the tree, the milk in the child, and thus are connected by a feedback loop.   In operant conditioning a conditioner simply steps in to manipulate the environment to manipulate the subject, thus simulating the process of reinforcement that otherwise occurs "naturally" or as circumstance or chance.

There are many refinements possible with the basic process. In teaching autistic children, a complex act such as getting one's hat from a peg and putting it on can be broken into many simpler acts--walking to the peg, reaching out, grasping the hat, putting it on--each one of which is positively reinforced.   In teaching large university classes, the learning process can be individualized by permitting each student to advance to the next level of complexity in problem-solving only after having mastered the previous level.   An entire ward of inmates in a mental institution could be conditioned by a token economy into becoming more self-sufficient.   New feelings of independence then might reinforce the desired behavior even further.   Used in these ways, operant conditioning would raise the same kinds of ethical questions that other methods of control do, but perhaps not so urgently.   The people being conditioned can still keep their wits about them. Their inner recesses aren't attacked as pervasively as with drugs and surgery.   Grinspoon and Singer, for example, suggest that conditioning programs for hyperactive children replace amphetamine use whenever possible:

> Behavior modification techniques, while they are no panacea
> and possess their own significant potential for abuse, do have
> this virtue: their proper application requires on the part of those
> who employ them a sensitivity to the needs, talents, and pref-
> erences of the individual child. Rather than simply making a

child more manageable, as drugs often do, such techniques may bring out his best qualities. Moreover, these techniques allow the child to discover his impulses and to make use of his own powers of self-control in dealing with them. They do not just abolish temporarily the more disturbing impulses, thereby rendering control unnecessary. Behaviors learned through the use of such techniques potentially can be generalized to many situations beyond the specific situation in which the behaviors were originally conditioned.... In contrast, drug-facilitated learning is not only not generalized to a broad spectrum of situations, but evidence suggests it is actually forgotten quite readily....[33]

But Skinner goes further. He builds on the discovery that more than instincts or habits change in conditioning. Along with new behavior come new attitudes; a child who no longer sucks his thumb _feels_ more secure; he doesn't need to be made to feel more secure as a prerequisite for ending the symptom of his insecurity. Cotter's study suggests that the inmates of his well-conditioned hospital felt better about themselves after being forced to work. Curiously, anxiety decreases as its _symptoms_ are changed; or to put it another way, the reward for acceptable behavior seems to lessen the strength of the stimulus for unacceptable behavior.

From this it follows that hypothetically all of a child's attitudes could be conditioned along with the child's behavior if operant conditioning were pervasive and efficient enough. Furthermore, the conditioner would need to shape a new feedback loop between subject and environment only at the beginning; once established, it would sustain itself; and if the conditioner worked scientifically enough so that Positive Reinforcement always followed predictably and consequently from Behavior, the relationship between subject and environment could become perfectly harmonious and predictable. Chance would evaporate; misunderstanding between two similarly conditioned subjects would become extremely unlikely.

In his most visionary works, Walden Two and Beyond Freedom and Dignity, as Skinner pursues this line of thought, behavior modification grows from a therapeutic or pedagogical technology into a sweeping program of social reform. His language echoes Delgado's as he discovers the same obstacles

to his vision: "The literature of freedom has given us a false
sense that men are truly autonomous creatures, each a world
of law unto himself." To the contrary: "The escape route of
[autonomy] is slowly closed as new evidences of the predictability
of human behavior are discovered. . . . By questioning the control exercised by autonomous man and demonstrating the control
exercised by the environment, a science of behavior also
seeks to question dignity or worth."[34] The literature of dignity
he goes on to say, gives humans credit for what they do beyond
the call of duty. It is irrelevant because humans do nothing
that is beyond the call of very complex stimuli.

Skinner thinks that the humanists' overfondness for a
belief in human independence causes them to want to leave much
to chance which could be controlled by behavior technologies.
Skinner dislikes accident as much as Delgado: "It is true that
accidents have been responsible for almost everything men have
achieved to date, and they will no doubt continue to contribute to
human accomplishment, but there is no virtue in an accident as
such. The unplanned always goes wrong.'[35] And like Delgado,
he recognized that to remake the social world by scientific means,
would be to make a world to suit a different kind of creature
than that which now calls itself human: "The problem is to design a world which will be liked not by people as they now are
but by those who live in it. . . . It would be liked because people
have been taught to like it, for reasons that do not always bear
scrutiny."[36]

Response to Skinner

John R. Platt sympathetically describes and defends all as-.
pects of Skinner's theory and practice. He compares Skinner
to Darwin, as equally important revolutionaries of social theory.
He describes in detail Skinner's techniques (in greater detail than
this review does) and cites its successful application in mental
hospitals. He distinguishes them from the "stereotyped Pavlo-
vian behavior methods in Brave New World": he explains how
Skinner is often misinterpreted by critics who fail to catch the
humanness and irony in his language.

But ironically when Platt admits the cogency of some of the
critical arguments against Skinner's broad social theory, and

sets out to "reconcile" them, he makes the same critical points himself. Platt's argument is that each human being is genetically distinct and grows up in a unique environment linked to him or her by a unique cybernetic feedback loop. Each person's pattern of conditioned responses is going to be different. Therefore his or her behavior is impossible to predict. Similar techniques of conditioning that will work for some won't work for all. Tailoring conditioning for each individual in a society would not be feasible because no conditioner could know enough. Platt coins a phrase for the resistant uniqueness:

> Private-indeterminacy simply means that your eye cannot see
> my sunbeam and your ear cannot be at this point of resonance,
> so you cannot know the private and ever-changing inputs of my
> initial state. The jailer, absolute in deterministic behavioral
> control may chain the prisoner to the wall, but he cannot see the
> cockroach--or the jailer--from the point of view that prisoner
> has. These complex and private operations determine each of
> our outcomes and behaviors in ways that no experimenter or
> controller can entirely measure or predict. If anyone still
> wishes to say that we are behaving deterministically "in prin-
> ciple, " he can; but it is operationally an empty statement if the
> prediction is, in principle, not possible itself because of in-
> complete information. And these unpredictable components of
> behavior could properly be called "self-determining" in the
> sense that they are reliable brain operations that are not being
> determined by anyone else.[37]

It is Skinner's failure to acknowledge this existential basis of each human experience, Platt says, that makes him miss the point of humanist critics such as Krutch, Maslow, and C. S. Lewis. These writers claim that Skinner's determinism ignores the unique contours of individual men in order to deal with them at a lower level where they all have very similar drives, fears, and desires. To work, Skinner's conditioning must first sim-plify the people to be conditioned.

When Skinner's theory is corrected by a sensitivity to the existential nature of man, Platt thinks that it gains a power to help individuals control themselves and cure themselves of unwanted habits. He quotes Saint Paul's cry of despair: "For the good that I would do I do not: but the evil which I would not, that I do, "[38] and suggests it need no longer be made. "Skinner's

method of designing reinforcers for self-control may be the
most important contribution to ethical practice in 2000 years. "[39]
But as Platt goes on to reconcile the behaviorist's position
with the humanist's position, he simply restates the first and
abandons the second. He begins to talk about how Skinner's
method could apply to the way a whole society shapes its moral
code to insure its survival. The old warrior codes that helped the
survival of tribes and small nation states are now worthless and
need replacement by a system of rewards and reinforcement for
the new values needed for survival in a complex world. Skinner's
technology would use positive reinforcement rather than negative
and thus phase out the practice of humanly inflicted pain in our
experience. As Platt argues this way, we are back again with
the problem of controlling people to change behavior molded by
a tremendous diversity of tradition and experience into more
rational and "simpler" behavior. Platt does acknowledge that
this line of thinking leads to an inevitable question: "Who is
going to prescribe and impose this more effective ethics on the
rest of us?" Skinner quotes C. S. Lewis as protesting: "...
The power of man to make himself what he pleases...means...
the power of some men to make other men what they please.
[Quoted by Skinner in Beyond Freedom and Dignity, p. 206.]
The answer is, as it has always been, that the controlling elites
are teachers, leaders, and officials whose methods and values
are accepted or adapted by the whole community."[40] But Platt
is not intimidated by this apparent invocation of an elitist social
theory. He considers his most telling point in the defense of
Skinner to be his reference to Skinner's means of preventing a
tyrannic leadership in his new community. Skinner would set
up a society in which important consequences would be brought
to bear on the behavior of the controller by those controlled.
Leaders and followers would reciprocally condition their behavior so that neither could get the upper hand. The trouble with the
checks and balances provided by the United States Constitution
in this regard is that they permit too much polarization and
hostility to exist after the necessary compromises are made.
Skinner's society would be more scientifically homogenous.
Hostility would be anticipated and defused. People would be
locked into a balanced world of universally acceptable values and
immediately achievable goals.

Who Plays God?

A skeptic could ask at this point who <u>outside</u> this integrated system would set it up to become self-sufficient. The skeptical Professor Burris in Skinner's novelistic <u>Walden Two</u> put the question this way to Frazier, the Skinnerian controller of a utopian community:

> "You mean you think you're God?" I said, deciding to get it over with.
> Frazier snorted in disgust.
> "I said there was a curious similarity, " he said.
> "Don't be absurd. "
> "No, really. The parallel is quite fascinating. Our friend Castle is worried about the conflict between long-range dictatorship and freedom. Doesn't he know he's merely raising the old question of predestination and free will? All that happens is contained in an original plan, yet at every stage the individual seems to be making choices and determining the outcome. The same is true of Walden Two. Our members are practically always doing what they want to do--what they 'choose' to do-- but we see to it that they will want to do precisely the things which are best for themselves and the community. Their behavior is determined, yet they're free.
> "Dictatorship and freedom--predestination and free will. " Frazier continued. "What are these but pseudo-questions of linguistic origin? When we ask what Man can make of Man, we don't mean the same thing by 'Man' in both instances. We mean to ask what a few men can make of mankind. And that's the all-absorbing question of the twentieth century. What kind of world can we build--those of us who understand the science of behavior?"
> "Then Castle was right. You're a dictator, after all. "
> "No more than God. Or rather less so. Generally, I've let things alone. I've never stepped in to wipe out the evil works of men with a great flood. Nor have I sent a personal emissary to reveal my plan and to put my people back on the track. The original design took deviations into account and provided automatic corrections. It's rather an improvement upon Genesis. "[41]

In a conversation with Skinner, Carl R. Rogers criticized the providential system of <u>Walden Two</u> precisely for its comprehen-

siveness. He sees no way for those within the system to change
it once the master plan has been set and the master has retired
from the scene:

> Thus if we chose as our goal the state of happiness for human
> beings (a goal deservedly ridiculed by Aldous Huxley in Brave
> New World), and if we involved all of society in a successful
> scientific program by which people became happy, we would be
> locked in a colossal rigidity in which no one would be free to
> question this goal, because our scientific operations could not
> transcend themselves to question their guiding purposes. And
> without laboring this point, I would remark that colossal rigid-
> ity, whether in dinosaurs or dictatorships, has a very poor re-
> cord of evolutionary survival. [42]

Roger's basic argument is that science cannot generate its
own values. German scientists working on guided missiles worked
just as energetically for Hitler as they later did for the United
States or Russia, depending on who captured them. Someone
always has to decide how a program will be used, and the decision will follow personal, ideological or arbitrary principles
at will. So there needs to be more than a few individuals deciding how a society should be run and, after it is running, how it
should adapt itself to changing conditions. Rogers suggests that
Skinner adopt for his system the goals John Dewey gave to education and that recent psychotherapy has adopted for its own--
the creation of many intelligent self-sufficient human individuals.
He quotes a statement of John Dewey's approvingly: "Science has
made its way by releasing, not by suppressing, the elements of
variation, of invention and innovation, of novel creation in individuals. "[43] Rogers concludes:

> I believe it is clear that such a view as I have been describing
> does not lead to any definable utopia. It would be impossible
> to predict its final outcome. It involves a step-by-step develop-
> ment based on a continuing subjective choice of purposes, which
> are implemented by the behavioral sciences. It is in the direc-
> tion of the "open society, " as that term has been defined by
> Popper where individuals carry responsibility for personal de-
> cisions. It is at the opposite pole from his concept of the closed
> society, of which Walden Two would be an example. [44]

In response to Rogers, Skinner reiterated his position (developed at length in his later book, Beyond Freedom and Dignity) that no such thing as a free individual exists anyway. The new goal of psychotherapy is chasing an illusion:

> What evidence is there that a client ever truly becomes truly self-directing? What evidence is there that he ever makes a truly inner choice of ideal or goal? Even though the therapist does not do the choosing, even though he encourages "self-actualization"—he is not out of control as long as he holds himself ready to step in when occasion demands—when, for example, the client chooses the goal of becoming a more accomplished liar or murdering his boss. But supposing the therapist does withdraw completely or is no longer necessary—what about all the other forces acting upon the client? Is the self-chosen goal independent of his early ethical and religious training? of the folk-wisdom of his group? of the opinions and attitudes of others who are important to him? Surely not. The therapeutic situation is only a small part of the world of the client. From the therapist's point of view it may appear to be possible to relinquish control. But the control passes, not to a "self," but to forces in other parts of the client's world.[45]

He repeats his plea that the pervasive fact of control be recognized so that human beings can set about becoming better at organizing their world:

> Fear of control, generalized beyond any warrant, has led to a misinterpretation of valid practices and the blind rejection of intelligent planning for a better way of life. In terms which I trust Rogers will approve, in conquering this fear we shall become more mature and better organized and shall, thus, more fully actualize ourselves as human beings.[46]

Other writers criticize Skinner by saying that insistence on ignoring human uniqueness might just cause it to disappear. Willard Gaylin thinks that Skinner ignores the radical unpredictability of human behavior, but fears that this lack would not necessarily make his program for social reform any less successful: "The principle that our view of man will create a man in that image seems a reasonable assumption. Psychological and sociological theories do become self-fulfilling prophecies, and this must be a consideration in any attempts to engineer a man. "47 Gaylin fears that in the process of "improving" man, Skinner would have to remove what is uniquely human about him: human unpredictability in a life of fascinating and terrible change. "In many ways we have been better served by happenstance than social design. One need only look at the state of our institutions today--our prisons, our mental institutions, and our schools-- to question the wisdom of social science in social engineering. "48

Robert Neville would add another item to the list of intolerable sacrifices Skinner's system would demand. He fears the loss, paradoxically, of a sense of loss:

> Perhaps the most important kind of personal freedom is the af-
> firmation of the value of life in the face of inevitable compromise
> and loss. A cheap way out in the conflict of values is to believe
> one side really does not count, or is secretly served by being
> subordinated to the other. The truth is, we must balance and
> choose with inevitable loss. A person who does this consciously,
> keen on both the success and sorrow, is free in possessing life
> realistically. A society that does that has nobility. Our society's
> failure to do that will mean that behavior control's vast powers
> will be deployed by custom, avarice, blind hope, and chance. 49

Gerald Leach, on the other hand, is inspired by the visions of Skinner and Delgado, and their promises to emancipate human life from ancient hobbles: "As Dr. José Delgado has put it, E. S. B. [Electrical Stimulation of the Brain] is beginning to make us realize that 'human behavior, happiness, good and evil, are after all, products of cerebral physiology....' And if this makes one feel degradingly like an electro-chemical puppet, I can only say that I prefer this feeling to the belief that I am controlled by wild devils in my head. "50

He himself doesn't fear that their programs will get out of hand to the point that they will crush human creative expression. Anyone who does, he says, should consider how similar dangers have been handled in the past: "One might ask why every government and population has overwhelmingly voted against an equally subtle and pernicious form of mind control--subliminal advertising. "51 But he finally seems a bit uneasy with any program of drugging or surgery or operant conditioning that would neglect what already lies in the hands of many of the individuals in today's world:

"If we all used a hundredth of the present body of knowledge about human psychology and motivation to modify behavior constructively and sensitively, we could do so much to realize the ancient dreams of human happiness. Chemical and electrical control of the brain may bring great changes, but they must only be aids to what we would accomplish by psychological and social change. After all, we are more than electro-chemical machines."52

Chapter 5

Death and Dying – New Criteria for Death, Heroic Medicine, Organ Transplants, and Euthanasia

The Cases

1   A 23-year-old unmarried miner is seriously injured in a
mine explosion. He loses both legs and part of a hand, and
suffers severe burns over half of his body. He is blinded and
made partially deaf. Soon after being admitted to a hospital, he
is sent to an intensive care unit. There he is placed in a special
"clean" room and made to lie perfectly still, except once a day
when his body is immersed in a chemical bath to protect his
skin from infection.

For one month the patient remains unaware of his surround-
ings. Gradually he gains a clear awareness of what is happening
to him and where he is. Despite heavy sedation he experiences
continual and intense pain. He inquires of his doctor his chances
of recovery and being released from the hospital. The doctor
tells him frankly that he can't make any predictions, but thinks
that the burns will require hospital care for the rest of the year,
and intensive home care for the rest of his life. The young man
thinks over his life for a few days, then asks the doctor to discontinue the chemical-bath therapy, knowing full well that without it he will surely soon die. He states that he has no family
responsibilities, and that he has no wish to live suffering as
a cripple. The doctor agrees to his request. He orders the
nurses in attendance to make the patient as comfortable as possible and to discontinue therapy.

The nurses, however, immediately complain to the hospital staff. The doctor is brought before the hospital ethics board.
He justifies his decision to the board by arguing that intensive
burn therapy cannot be considered ordinary or required when a
patient doesn't consent to it. The board overrules his argument

and decision to discontinue therapy. They argue that a therapy
that doesn't endanger a patient's life cannot be considered extraordinary and that no patient has a right to avoid therapy he
needs to sustain his life, whatever its quality or misery.

2   A young woman is struck by a car one evening while stum-
bling across a city street. The first policeman to arrive on the
scene discovers that her heart has stopped beating and that she
isn't breathing. He smells liquor on her mouth and clothes. He
applies mouth-to-mouth resuscitation and heart massage. When
an ambulance arrives she is immediately placed on a portable
respirator and taken to an emergency ward where she is attached
to a larger machine. Physicians examine her and discover that
she has suffered massive brain damage. Her electroencephalogram is isoelectric (flat). But she does have mild reflex reactions
to painful stimuli. They diagnose that the neocortex has been
destroyed but the brain stem which controls certain reflexive
functions still lives. When they turn off the respirator for a few
minutes they discover that the woman is unable to breathe spontaneously. She is put back on the machine. Her blood continues
to circulate, her lungs to ventilate.

After the diagnosis is made, her husband is contacted by
phone and asked to come to the hospital. The doctors explain
to him that there is no hope for her recovery as a functional
human being, but that she is not yet medically dead. She could
live on in her present state on the machine for an indefinite
period of time. If the respirator were turned off, however, all
her vital functions would stop within about five minutes. She
is only artificially alive; she is "naturally" dead. They ask his
permission to turn off the machines and to be permitted to transplant her healthy heart into another young woman in the hospital
dying of heart disease. The husband consents saying, "Sure,
at least this way she'll be good for something. Otherwise she's
just a dead drunk." He signs the consent form. She is declared
dead, taken off the machines, and has her heart removed.

3   An elderly man very close to death from cancer contracts
pneumonia. He has previously told his physician that he wants
him to use any means to keep him alive as long as possible.
When the physician hears of his current state of health, however,

he orders that no antibiotics be given. Instead the patient is
given a mild sedative. Several days later he dies of pneumonia.

The Issues: New Kinds of Dying

Black's Law Dictionary defines death as: "The cessation of
life, the ceasing to exist; defined by physicians as a total stop-
page of the circulation of the blood, and a cessation of the animal
and vital functions consequent thereupon, such as respiration,
pulsation, etc." The special feature of this legal definition is
that it corresponds more or less to the popular conception of
death. Traditionally when a person stopped breathing and the
pulse stopped he or she was thought dead, whether the observer
was a friend, a family member, a policeman on the street,
or a physician in a hospital. The tests a doctor would run would
differ only slightly in sophistication from the popular tests of a
feather or a mirror placed over the mouth.

Modern medical science has made this definition obsolete.
Now, hooked up to machines, the blood and lungs needn't stop
functioning even if the patient lies comatose and cannot breathe
on his own. If such a body is continually ventilated and supplied
with the nourishment of intravenous feeding it can even continue
to metabolize. It remains warm, supple, and indistinguishable
from a person in a deep sleep, even though the sleep might be
permanent. The machines thus create a semblance of life that
can no longer be carefully distinguished from traditionally
understood states of life or death.

Maintained in such a state for a time, a patient can rally back
to life. Gerald Leach cites the case of a young boy who fell into
a partly frozen Norwegian river and who was trapped underwater
for twenty-two minutes. When taken from the water his skin
was blue, his eyes dilated, and there was no pulse or heartbeat.
Spontaneous heartbeat and breathing commenced after two and a
half hours of mouth-to-mouth respiration, heart massages,
drug injections and blood transfusions. Five times during the
next twenty-four hours, his breathing stopped and was started
again by an artificial respirator. Within ten days he had recovered progressively until he was able to recognize his parents.
Then he fell into a deep coma for five weeks with no noticeable
brain function. After the seventh week he revived and within

six months was almost totally recovered except for some
clumsy finger movements and a reduced area of vision. [1]

In other cases there are good reasons why someone might
want to turn the machines off. They are expensive to run, and
would seem senseless to run if the patient couldn't possibly
recover a conscious, independent life. Another patient might
be able to use the organs if they could be transplanted from a
declared cadaver. Perhaps more importantly, a person should
be provided the decency of a <u>natural death</u> and a burial in the
presence of relations and friends. In a celebrated case, Joseph
Quinlan asked that the respirators keeping his daughter Karen
"alive" in a deep coma be turned off "so that we could place her
body and soul in the tender loving hands of the Lord."

Physicians have recently redefined the cessation of life to
fit the new kinds of life and death available on the machines. The
criteria of the Ad Hoc Committee of the Harvard Medical School
to Examine the Definition of Brain Death look past the heart and
lungs to the brain for irreversible coma: "a total unawareness
to externally applied stimuli and inner need and complete un-
responsiveness." This state can be tested for even while the
patient breathes on a machine by checking the patient's reactions
to light shone in the eyes, loud noises, and painful stimulation
of the muscles and nerves. If there is no groan, withdrawal of
a limb, or quickening of respiration, it could be assumed that
the brain is no longer functioning. "Irreversible coma with
abolition of central nervous system activity is evidenced in part
by the absence of elicitable reflexes." After performing these
tests attending physicians can confirm their diagnosis using an
electroencephalogram (EEG) machine to measure brain activity. An isoelectric or flat EEG would support the external
indications that the neocortex and the brain stem were dead
beyond recall. The tests are repeated in twenty-four hours.
If there is still no sign of brain activity, then the patient is
declared dead <u>before</u> the machines are turned off, to free the
physician from feelings or legal accusations that he had killed
a living patient. The criteria end with a qualification: "The
validity of such data as indications of irreversible cerebral
damage depends on the exclusion of two conditions: hypothermia
(temperature below 90 f. 32.2 C) or central nervous system
depressants such as barbiturates." [2]

The Crux of the Problem with the "New" Death

However these criteria might clarify the use of respirators for physicians, assuage their consciences, and protect them from malpractice suits, they do not work to make life and death on the machine any less strange for the layperson. No layperson would be expected to understand how to test for complex reflexive reaction, much less be able to interpret an electroencephalogram (which is only used to confirm the earlier tests). None would be likely to get the chance, either. These tests would be run on patients in hospitals involved in very different kinds of dying than those at home or on a battlefield or at the scene of an accident, as other fields of medical science labor more and more successfully to deliver patients to intensive care units to die.

The Harvard report itself acknowledges the extraordinary nature of the technology that its authors wish to help regulate. It quotes and concurs with the statement of Pope Pius XII that it is not obligatory to continue to use extraordinary means indefinitely in hopeless cases. But the report thereby implies that there appears to be some obligation to use extraordinary means if the case is not hopeless. As the committee sets about determining when the second case becomes the first, their criteria implicitly support the use of the machines which made them necessary, and so comply with the increasing alienation of clinical death from what has been traditionally perceived as "natural dying."

Organ transplant technology can make the process even more strange. The most successful transplants work with fresh organs from bodies declared dead only minutes before the organs are removed, and so can make efficient use of both the new machines and the new criteria for death. Paul Ramsey cites the case of a patient on a respirator flown to a distant transplant center along with members of her family. Upon arrival at the clinic she was declared dead in an area adjacent to an operating room where another patient lay awaiting a transplanted heart. The possibility arises that a potential donor could be declared technically dead too fast for the comfort or understanding of the surviving family and kin, then cut up and given away; the process could scar the living so deeply that no medicine could

cure its harm. Contemporary writing on the ethics of dying
considers the new ways of dying in light of the traditions of
death in order to find some ways of combining them for the comfort of living mortals.

Criticisms of the New Criteria

Medical researchers have discovered practical problems with
the Harvard criteria: problems which raise ethical questions
about the quality of life that the machines maintain. There is
evidence that cardiac arrest might destroy a patient's neocortex
but not the lower areas of the brain; on a respirator the patient
might respond to reflex-stimuli and, after some time, begin
to breathe spontaneously, even though there is no possibility
whatsoever that the patient will ever regain consciousness. A
team headed by J. B. Brierley concluded a study of two such
cases who survived more than five months on a respirator
(they cite another case where the patient lived for twenty-seven
months):

> ...According to the criteria...both the present patients would
> be regarded as "alive" although the neurophysiological assess-
> ment, made during life, that the neocortex was dead in each,
> was confirmed by the neuropathological examinations.
>   These two cases...may be regarded as products of the pres-
> ent era of intensive care and they may not long remain unique.
> Their documentation in clinical and neuropathological terms
> represents a challenge to any definition of life that is unconcerned
> with the functional and structural integrity of the neocortex.[3]

The higher functions of the brain are those, the researchers
also point out, that demarcate man from the lower primates and
all other vertebrates and invertebrates. The Harvard criteria
thus can make no assessment of the quality of life.

Robert Morison fears that doctors might use the criteria to
fend off the responsibility of judging whether certain kinds of
lives on the machine might not fall seriously short of being
worth living. Maintaining the technical life of a cardiac patient,
for example, could drain the resources of the family, occupy
medical facilities that could be better used for patients with
better prospects, and could deny the use of organs for trans-

plants for critically long periods. Instead of applying them too
strictly, doctors should be free to determine when the "whole"
human being has ceased to function as a whole:

> Whatever the metaphors are used to describe the situation,
> it is clear that it is the complex interactions that make the
> characteristic human being. The appropriate integration of
> these interactions is only loosely coupled to the physiological
> functions of circulation and respiration. The latter continue for
> a long time after the integrated "personality" has disappeared.
> Conversely, the natural rhythms of heart and respiration can
> fail, while the personality remains intact. The complex human
> organism does not often fail as a unit....
>
> Squirm as we may to avoid the inevitable, it seems time to
> admit to ourselves that there is simply no hiding place and that
> we must shoulder the responsibility of deciding to act in such a
> way as to hasten the declining trajectories of some lives, while
> doing our best to slow down the decline of others. And we have
> to do this on the basis of some judgement on the quality of the
> lives in question. [4]

He fears that the same doctors that routinely hook patients up to
a respirator will routinely leave them there until brain death
occurs, regardless of circumstances.

In a following article in the same journal, Leon R. Kass replies that such a decision "to hasten the declining trajectories
of some lives" would be ethical only if it were made solely for
the benefit of the patient. The trouble with most quality-of-life
arguments, he feels, is that they actually substitute an economic
analysis for medical criteria with the result that the patient is
still considered something of an object whose value or functioning
could be grafted. He reasons that the expenses to the family or
the insurance company, or the needs of a transplant team must
have no part in determining when a patient should be allowed to
die. Even if a patient dies in parts, there is some point at which
the wholeness of life is lost irrevocably. Only when that point
is reached should the patient be allowed to die for his own good. [5]
Whatever their disagreements, both writers share the view that
the existence of technical or artificial life should never be
equated with a life necessarily worth living.

Hans Jonas fears the criteria's proviso that the patient shall
be declared dead <u>before</u> the machines are turned off. This might
lead to permitting experimentation with a new type of "living"

cadaver. He reasons that the new definition does not draw a
clear demarcation between life and death, and so one cannot use
it to dismiss out of hand the ancient and enduring idea that death
occurs when breathing and pulsing cease. The artificially supported condition of the comatose patient is still therefore a kind
of life, however reduced. "In this state of marginal ignorance
and doubt the only course is to lean over backward toward the
side of possible life. It follows that interventions such as I
described shall be regarded as vivisection and on no account be
performed on a human body in that equivocal and threshold condition." So long as the body "still breathes, pulses and functions
otherwise [it] must still be considered a residual continuance of
the subject that loved and was loved."[6]

Jonas argues further that this new emphasis on the death of the
brain as opposed to the death of the body reminds him of the old
body-soul dualism. Both ignore or slight the bodily identity of
an individual human, as unique and expressive as speech itself.
"How else could a man love a woman and not merely her brains?"[7]

David D. Rutstein suspects that the criteria are designed
simply to facilitate organ transplants. Declaring the patient
dead before turning off the machines is not so much to protect
the conscience of the doctor as to allow the organs to stay fresh
until they are taken out. He shares Jonas's view that the criteria
could be used to insert death beds into assembly lines.[8]

A Defense of the New Criteria

The Task Force on Death and Dying of the Institute of Society,
Ethics and Life Sciences set about laying fears of this sort
to rest in a sympathetic appraisal of the new criteria.[9] They
recognize four areas of concern: the vagueness of the definition
of death (the criteria assess that death has occurred, not precisely
when it has occurred); the fear that the new criteria are primarily intended to facilitate transplants; mistrust of new powers
vested in the attending physician; and fears that the new definition will lend itself to updating at an increasing risk to the dignity of the dying patient. They respond to each concern in turn,
in essence arguing that the Harvard report makes very clear
distinctions between the questions of clinical death which it
considers and the questions about the quality of life which it
does not.

They argue that the new criteria really posit no new definition of death, but rather refine an alternative means for detecting the same "old" phenomenon of death. They reason furthermore that the Harvard report takes pains to separate the question of when a patient is dead from the question of when treatment
should be withdrawn to allow the patient to die. The report
approvingly quotes the statement of Pope Pius XII that in certain cases extraordinary life support needn't be continued. The
task force agrees with the committee that the two questions
should be kept separate.

The task force argues that the criteria do not exhaustively
regulate organ transplant technology. Other ethical norms
govern this procedure, such as the usual requirement that the
dying patient's physician not be a member of the transplant team,
and that he or she declare a patient dead independently of the
team's needs. A similar defense could be made against Jonas's
argument that new forms of experimentation would now be possible. The ethics governing human experimentation would come
into play.

The task force also defends the criteria against critics who
fear that the criteria might be updated. The EEG which is used
to confirm the tests for reflexes, it is often feared, might
eventually be used to determine death itself. They refer to
work of Brierley which proves that the lower brain and the
functions it controls might survive the death of the neocortex
represented by a flat EEG. They point out that the report
explicitly states that the EEG is to have a secondary role: "To
prevent... confusion and the possible dangerous practices that
might result from a shift to exclusive reliance on the EEG we
urge that the clinical and more comprehensive criteria of the
Harvard Report be adopted. "[10]

Their defense of the criteria is more equivocal, however,
when they take up the criticism that the new definition of death
puts the defining and declaring power exclusively in the judgment of the doctor. They argue that to avoid confusion and
malpractice, the law should conform uniformly to updated medical opinion. Even Black's definition includes the phrase
"defined by physicians. " But the task force acknowledges there
is cause for concern from the fact that until recently the physician's definition and the popular one were for all practical pur-

poses the same while the physician's definition could now lead
to practices which might confuse or horrify the community.
There is a need to air the new definition in the community in
order to gain public acceptance and for the legal protection of
physicians:

> We are sympathetic to the value of having any changes in the
> concept of death, or even major changes in criteria for de-
> termining death, ratified by the community, as a sign of public
> acceptance and for the legal protection of physicians. On the
> other hand, we are concerned about the possibility of confused,
> imprecisely drafted, or overly rigid statutes. Moreover, we
> do not believe that legislation is absolutely necessary in order
> to permit physicians to use the new criteria, once these re-
> ceive the endorsement and support of the medical profession.
> Clearly, these matters of decision-making and the role of law
> need further and widespread discussion.[11]

The task force tends to see the educational process as a one-
way street; the doctors educate the public to the new values
and procedures.

Remaining Doubts: The Powers Given to Doctors by the Criteria

The danger in this, according to some writers, is that the
doctors who use and promulgate this pragmatic or clinical
definition of death to affect the way they declare death, and
more critically, treat the dying, might not be sympathetic to
the sway which the sacred, mythic power of death holds over
mortal minds. Certain doctors simply aren't sympathetic.
Walter S. Ross comments: "In my opinion, death is an insult:
the stupidest, ugliest thing that can happen to a human being....
When a doctor says a patient is beyond help, he's really admitting
his lack of willingness to fight. Some say we prolong life too
often. But the people whose lives are prolonged don't say that.
It's always the healthy survivors who insist on the patient's
right to die with dignity."[12]   Dr. David Karnofsky defends the
use of "aggressive or extraordinary means of treatment" to prolong life even when the state of dying may often be protracted
by "expensive and desperate supportive measures." He views

the frequent pleas of state planners, efficiency experts, social workers, philosophers, theologians, economists, and humanitarians that moribund patients be allowed to die quickly, without pain and with dignity as often being tantamount to a cowardly desire to sweep away "the inevitable debris of life." The medical imperative demands that the physician carry on heroically until the issue is taken out of his hands.[13]   Both Ross and Karnofsky are typical of doctors who could use the Harvard criteria as the only outside limit they would accept to the vigorous application of heroic medicine to either a conscious or unconscious terminal patient.

Philosophers and the public might have reason to criticize these attitudes, their contention being not necessarily with the validity of the criteria as such, but with the manner in which they are used to regulate heroic medicine for the dying. It is a question of ethical style. At the same time, they would tend to see the new criteria for death and the use of heroic medicine as related issues in practice, whatever the sincere claim of the committee and the task force that the intent of the report was to separate them in the abstract.

Some psychologists suspect that doctors might tend to use heroic medicine indiscriminately because they fear death excessively. Herman Feifel in a study of doctors' attitudes towards death discovered them to be significantly more afraid of death than either healthy or sick people in control groups: "Interestingly although the overwhelming majority of physicians wanted to be informed if they had an incurable disease, they were less willing than the patients to provide such information to others in the same boat."[14]   The study speculates that the physician selects his or her occupational role for varying reasons, among them to help control personal concerns about death. When unsettled by a dying patient or an emotionally distraught family, "his reawakened anxieties about death may lead him to unwittingly disinherit his patient psychologically at the very time he enhances attention to his physiological needs."[15]   It would be well within this speculation to believe that a doctor's fear of death might lead him or her to put off telling a patient of a terminal illness, and then to use the impersonal means of heroic medicine to cope with his or her own anxiety rather than the patient's real needs.

Donald Oken, M. D., did another study on how doctors handle
terminal cancer patients and also discovered that they tend to
tell patients as little as possible about their condition while
desiring to be told the straight facts themselves if they should
become terminally ill. The inconsistency is characteristic,
Oken says, of emotionally determined attitudes. He comes to
conclusions similar to Feifel's:

> Among the motivations for entering medicine, the wish to
> conquer suffering and death stands high on the list. Practicing
> physicians are not the kind of persons who can sit quietly by
> while nature pursues its course. One of the hardest things for
> a fledgling medical student to learn is watchful waiting. Few
> situations are as frustrating as sitting by impotently and "help-
> lessly" in the face of illness. Fatal illness is felt as a major
> defeat.[16]

Ivan Illich sees this fear developing out of the evolution of
myths about medicine since the middle ages. As medicine has
become more mechanized and more universally accessible, its
continuing failure to find a cure for death itself makes its practitioners anxious, prone to subconsciousness motivation. Hold-
ing off death increasingly becomes subconsciously the primary
goal of medicine, often to the neglect of more realistic, simpler,
and more reassuring comfort of the afflicted. There is an underlying assurance that if heroic medicine fails to banish death, at
least it dispenses a new uniform death under clinical conditions
for the old multifaceted kinds of dying. With this maturation
ritualized behavior substitutes for individualized care: all dying
patients are put on machines; all are declared dead by universally
accepted norms.
The rituals of heroic medicine, as do all rituals, Illich says,
hide a contradiction:

> In modern societies two contradictory concepts of death are
> simultaneously held....As a productive industry medicine is
> organized like an agency for the defense of mankind against a
> host of evil deaths, while as a world-wide ritual it is structured
> to foster the belief that natural extinction from peaceful exhaustion
> is the birthright of all men.
>   The ritual nature of modern health procedures hides from
> doctors and patients the contradiction between the ideal of a

natural death of which they want to die, and the reality of a
clinical death in which most contemporary men actually end.[17]

William May fears the consequences of a society flying in the
face of deeply rooted feelings about death. When a human being
feels the coming loss of his control over his flesh, he or she
feels the terrible loss of control over the world, the ability to
express the self with the body, and the loss of the sustaining
community. Heroic medicine could intensify rather than alleviate the sense of loss. Hoses and gadgets restrict movement,
clinical conditions replace all the colorful diversity of life,
doctors and family treat the patient with diffidence, fear, and
silence.

In the service of saving life, heroic medicine can sometimes
only assure that its final moments will be as miserable as possible. "...Our humanity is tested and revealed in the way in
which we behave toward death; by the same token, it is obscured
and diminished when death is concealed from view--when the dying
are forced to make their exit anonymously, their ending unwit-
nessed, uncherished, unsuffered, and unrecorded except in the
hospital files."[18]

Integrations

Other writers who share May's respect for the sacral process
of dying as well as a respect for modern medicine's powers for
resisting death have attempted to devise practical guidelines
for bringing them into balance. Paul Ramsey would not have a
doctor declare a patient dead until after the machines have been
turned off and it was clear that no spontaneous breathing or blood
circulation occurred. "No matter how fine the tests for telling
death, some stroke or brain damaged patients are going to get
through the net and must be declared to be still living."[19]   For
him the criteria would serve a more limited purpose than declaring death; they could be used to indicate the probability that
if the machines were turned off no natural functions would be
restored. Thus they would indicate that a patient was "dying,"
not dead, and still in need of care.

Ramsey also devotes a great deal of thought to what kind of
care all dying patients should enjoy. He thinks one should always

keep in mind the primary distinction between extraordinary and
ordinary means of care. Doctors tend to make the distinction
in terms of the state of the art; if a machine is effective and
widely distributed, its use is ordinary. A moralist, on the other
hand, tends to make the distinction in terms of the patient's
particular medical condition. If the patient is irrevocably dying,
all means to slow the process should be well considered extraordinary. Ramsey would make even further distinctions, following the lead of a moral theologian, Gerald Kelly, S. J. He is
willing to remove "ordinary" means under certain circumstances
from the class of morally or medically imperative means:

> Agreeing with those moralists who regard intravenous feed-
> ing as in itself an ordinary means (and who therefore judged it
> to be imperative), Kelly says instead that, "even granted that
> it is ordinary one may not immediately conclude that it is ob-
> ligatory. " An ordinary means may be out of place because of
> the condition of a patient--as out of place as unusual or heroic
> procedures.
>
> His argument is quite sufficient to make it unnecessary to
> distinguish between natural and artificial remedies in morally
> evaluating whether they should be used or not.[20]

In Ramsey's view, the moralist is thus free of any medical
imperative to preserve life at all cost. He would, if he adopted
Ramsey's principles, even be able to condone consensual
euthanasia:

> Never abandon care of the dying except when they are ir-
> retrievably inaccessible to human care, Never hasten the dying
> process except when it is entirely indifferent to the patient
> whether his dying is accomplished by an intravenous bubble of
> air or by the withdrawal of useless ordinary natural remedies
> such as nourishment. . . .
>
> Always keep officious treatments away from the dying in
> order to draw close to them in companying with them and car-
> ing for them; never, therefore, take positive action to usher them
> out of our presence or to hasten their departure from the human
> community, unless there is a kind of prolonged dying in which
> it is medically impossible to keep severe pain at bay.[21]

It would appear from Michael T. Sullivan's review of the
legal literature on the subject of care for the dying that Ramsey's

moralist would be thinking differently from most physicians and ahead of the present law, although in a direction Sullivan thinks the law should go. He cites cases in which, despite medical opposition, an elderly woman was allowed to refuse life-prolonging surgery; a young woman Jehovah's Witness was allowed to refuse life-saving blood transfusions on religious grounds. He cites another in which, in line with medical opposition, a court denied a young couple permission to refuse blood transfusions for their young child. He cites still other cases in which the court upheld the doctor's or hospital's presumption that they could control the method of a patient's dying, having left no alternatives to the individual himself.[22]

He argues that the individual should be allowed to control his personal relationships and the style of his dying as much as possible; if the patient is incompetent, a proctor should be appointed who could best protect his special interests. He concludes:

> The law's failure to recognize the dying person's rights, the dichotomy and confusion of case law regarding persons who have religious convictions about medical treatment, the officious assumption of authority over people's death style by professionals --all point to a pressing need for state legislation.
>
> This need now takes on huge proportions by swelling public rejection of death-taboo hypocrisy, by public recognition that death is as much a part of life as birth and by public insistence that the individual regain hegemony over his death-style.
>
> The writer does not believe legislation definitive of "death" is advisable in the context of this paper. The individual should decide whether he will employ the Harvard criteria, or some other definition for his death. And for reasons stated the living will is an inappropriate subject for legislation.
>
> The writer suggests the following:
> 1) statutory declaration that the constitutional right securative of life encompasses the individual's right within lawful means to choose his path of death;
> 2) statutory creation of a proctorship to insure enforcement of the individual's right to prescribe his death style, particularly
>   a) relationship with physicians, clergy, hospitals, nurses, para-professionals, and family;
>   b) death definition and organ donations;
>   c) funeral directions.[23]

Passive Euthanasia

Euthanasia literally means a "good death, " but has usually
been used in a more restricted sense to refer to mercy killing,
or putting moribund patients out of their misery by an injection
of air or a heavy dose of a sedative. Ramsey argues that if a
patient consented, it should be permitted if it would help him or
her toward a good dying, a dignified death. This kind of euthanasia is different from one imposed by a physician who makes an
independent judgment to kill a suffering patient. Such a practice would be much less acceptable if drugs were readily available to relieve the suffering of the dying person. Death then
could take its own time without causing undue misery.

[But the main focus of his arguments is in favor of a new kind
of euthanasia that can be viewed as an alternative to heroic
medicine. It could be called "passive" or "negative" euthanasia:
simply letting people die a comfortable natural death with or
without their explicit consent without postponement. Modern
respirators create this option; they shouldn't be allowed to preclude it.]

George Fletcher would agree that consent should rule whenever possible in such cases, even if a patient demanded of his
physician that he or she do everything to keep breathing going:
"If the doctor agrees to this bizarre demand, he becomes obligated to keep the respirator going indefinitely. " But more
often patients don't make their specific desires known, and
doctors don't ask. The question is a delicate one. In such
cases:

> The doctor's duty to prolong life is a function of his relation-
> ship with his patient; and in the typical case, that relationship
> devolves into the patient's expectations of the treatment he will
> receive. Those expectations, in turn, are a function of the
> practices prevailing in the community at the time, and prac-
> tices in the use of respirators to prolong life are no more and
> no less than what doctors actually do in the time and place.
> Thus, we have come full circle. We began the inquiry by ask-
> ing: Is it legally permissible for doctors to turn off respirators
> used to prolong the life of doomed patients? And the answer
> after our tortuous journey is simply: It all depends on what
> doctors customarily do. The law is sometimes no more pre-
> cise than that. [24]

In other words, doctors and patients (or laypeople) must talk together to define and adjust "common practice." The law can't make fine enough distinctions to be binding in every case.

Fletcher's reasoning shares the view of the statement adopted by the American Medical Association House of Delegates in 1913. It condemned mercy killing ("positive" euthanasia) but did say that "the cessation of the employment of extraordinary means to prolong the life of the body when there is irrefutable evidence that biological death is imminent is the decision of the patient and/or his immediate family. The advice and judgement of the physician should be freely available to the patient and/or his immediate family."[25]

The Karen Quinlan Case

The limitation of the law in this regard until the recent New Jersey Supreme Court decision becomes obvious in the celebrated case of Karen Quinlan, a young woman who had been lying in a deep coma for some time, kept alive by a respirator. According to the Harvard criteria, she was not dead; her EEG showed some minimal brain stem activity. Her parents, however, asked that the respirator be turned off so that she could die a natural death. Her doctors refused, saying that she was not dead and they had an obligation to keep her alive. On 10 November 1975, the presiding judge, Robert Muir, ruled that the doctors had the right in this case to decide. He reasoned that doctors are experts at the determination of death, are obligated to do everything humanly possible to sustain life, and are the final arbitrators of the best interests of the incompetent patient:

> There is a higher standard, a higher duty, that encompasses the uniqueness of human life, the integrity of the medical profession and the attitude of society. A patient is placed, or places himself in the care of a physician with the expectation that he (the physician) will do everything that is known to modern medicine, to protect the patient's life. He will do all within his human power to favor life against death.[26]

Judge Muir echoes Ross and Karnofsky and rejects the line of reasoning used by Sullivan and Fletcher in assigning the deciding voice in the discussion over the ethics of dying solely to the physician.

A lawyer commenting on the decision in a special section of a Hastings Center Report points out that the court could respond in no other way. Given a choice between restricting or permitting a mercy killing, it had to rule to protect life:

> Harsh as this may sound to those who are concerned more
> with immediate sympathetic relief for an anguished family than
> with the hazardous potential consequences of such a merciful
> action for thousands of defenseless incompetents in the future,
> the deeper instincts of the law were right in this case. For if
> legal guardians are allowed to judge the worth and viability of
> human life, then we should not be surprised to see many "mercy
> killings" of newborn defectives, retardates, genetically handi-
> capped, senile, and feeble-minded persons whose lives could
> end under liberalized involuntary euthanasia rulings.[27]

In other commentaries on the case, in the same issue of the Report, Melvin D. Levine states that "turning off ventilatory assistance is a common occurrence in medical centers...." He sees the danger of Muir's decision as that it might make doctors more reluctant to turn respirators on in the future, for fear of not being allowed to follow their best judgment or the wishes of the patient or guardian to turn them off again. "Ironically, then, discouraging physicians from disconnecting respirators might tend to a marked increase in passive euthanasia."[28] Paul Ramsey reiterates his position that a careful distinction must be made between ordinary and extraordinary medical care. The way the issue will be decided in each case would depend on the specifics of the case, but the discussion would have some objective goal. Trying to ascertain "ordinary" and therefore obligatory care would rule out the prior prejudices of the physician or the patient about mercy killing. The issue is rather the proper care of the dying. Alexander Capron fears "the opinion may even alter official notions of the proper relationship between doctors and patients and of what health care is all about--is it a human enterprise focused around the care of ailing persons or an elaborate system for developing and applying medical technology?"[29]

The Supreme Court of New Jersey, in repealing Judge Muir's decision in a ruling issued 31 March 1976, drew on the kinds of arguments The Hastings Center Report advanced, especially

those espoused by Ramsey and Capron. The court admitted that
according to the standards of the Ad Hoc Committee of Harvard
Medical College, Karen was not dead. Her lower brain was
still alive and permitting basic reflexes such as blinking and
swallowing to occur. (Her case is similar to those cited above
by J. B. Brierley where patients could live on for years in a
vegetative state with no hope for the recovery of their cognitive
or "higher brain" functions.) Furthermore, Judge Muir was
correct in deciding to accept the prevailing medical practice in
cases like this as the norm. Usually the practice is to continue
respiration until brain death occurs. But the New Jersey
Supreme Court also pointed out that in certain cases they judge
to be analogous, physicians customarily decide not to resusci-
tate terminal patients dying of painful and hopeless diseases
such as cancer. They have the good of the patient in view.
From this the court argues that if Karen Quinlan herself were
to become miraculously lucid, she could be permitted to decide
not to be resuscitated if and when she slipped back into a hopeless, comatose state. Her case is not like those in which patients are forced because of the state's interest in their welfare
to undergo treatment which promises to return them to health:

> We think that the State's interest contra weakens and the individ-
> ual's right to privacy grows as the degree of the bodily invasion
> increases and the prognosis dims. Ultimately there comes a
> point at which the individual's rights overcome the State interest.
> It is for that reason that we believe Karen's choice, if she were
> competent to make it, would be vindicated by the law. Her
> prognosis is extremely poor, -- she will never resume cognitive
> life. And the bodily invasion is very great, -- she requires
> 24 hour intensive nursing care, antibiotics, the assistance of a
> respirator, a catheter and feeding tube.[30]

Barring her impossible recovery, however, her family and
most specifically her father acting as guardian should be allowed
to make the decision for her, in consultation with sympathetic
and responsible physicians. The court expresses a wish that
in the future physicians "diffuse" their heavy responsibility in
such cases, that the prevailing medical practice have physicians
consulting with their colleagues and with the patient's family.
Their goal should be to define the difference between obligatory

"ordinary" treatment and "extraordinary" voluntary treatment
in specific cases. In addition to helping all concerned reach
a mutually acceptable decision, it would "free physicians, in
the pursuit of their healing vocation, from possible contamination
by self-interest or self-protection concerns which would inhibit
their independent medical judgments for the well being of their
dying patients."[31]

In conclusion, the court granted Joseph Quinlan guardianship
of his daughter and the right to choose for her other physicians
more sympathetic to his point of view. They declare further:

> Upon the concurrence of the guardian and family of Karen,
> should the responsible attending physicians conclude that there
> is no reasonable possibility of Karen's ever emerging from her
> present comatose condition to a cognitive, sapient state and
> that the life-support apparatus now being administered to Karen
> should be discontinued, they shall consult with the hospital
> "Ethics Committee" or like body of the institution in which Karen
> is then hospitalized. If that consultative body agrees that there
> is no reasonable possibility of Karen's ever emerging from her
> present comatose condition to a cognitive, sapient state, the
> present life-support system may be withdrawn and said action
> shall be without any civil or criminal liability therefore on the
> part of any participant, whether guardian, physician, hospital
> or others.[32]

Learning from the Dying

The subtitle of Elisabeth Kübler-Ross's book, On Death and
Dying, indicates whose voices she thinks should have the most
authority in any discussion on dying: "What the Dying Have
to Teach Doctors, Nurses, Clergy and Their Own Families."

> Is our concentration on equipment, on blood pressure, our
> desperate attempt to deny the impending death which is so
> frightening and discomforting to us that we displace all our
> knowledge into machines, since they are less close to us than
> the suffering face of another human being which would remind
> us once more of our lack of omnipotence, our own limits and
> failures, and last but not least perhaps our own mortality?
>   Maybe the question has to be raised: Are we becoming less
> human or more human? Though this book is in no way meant

to be judgmental, it is clear that whatever the answer may be, the patient is suffering more--not physically, perhaps, but emotionally. And his needs have not changed over the centuries, only our ability to gratify them.[33]

Her attentiveness to the dying as a psychiatrist has led to her discovery of five stages or different experiences in the act of prolonged dying. In the first stage, the patient denies that he or she is dying. Death has been feared so long that its approach is unbearable. In the second stage, the patient becomes very angry that death has arbitrarily decided to come before life is no longer worth living. This leads to the third stage, in which the patient begins to bargain with the doctor or with God for more time, promising increased devotion to a medical or moral regime. When the bargaining seems to fail, the patient becomes very depressed and feels defeated by the whole process beyond his or her control. Finally, if the patient is permitted to grope and grow through these stages, there can come a tranquil acceptance of fate that opens up a quiet and natural death to the dying and to all around affected by it. These progressive stages require, of course, that the patient be told he or she is dying with whatever sensitive indirection may be required, and that the use of machinery not be allowed to interfere with the progress of death, especially with the last stage of acceptance. Machines and assaultive medicine could force false hope where calm acceptance should be:

> Those who have the strength and the Love to sit with a dying patient in the silence that goes beyond words will know that this moment is neither frightening nor painful, but a peaceful cessation of the functioning of the body. Watching a peaceful death of a human being reminds us of a falling star; one of the millions of lights in a vast sky that flares up for a brief moment only to disappear into the endless night forever. To be a therapist to a dying patient makes us aware of the uniqueness of each individual in this vast sea of humanity. It makes us aware of our finiteness, our limited lifespan. Few of us live beyond our three score and ten years and yet in that brief time most of us create and live a unique biography and weave ourselves into the fabric of human history.[34]

Cadaver Organ Transplants

Organ transplant technology developed separately from heroic medicine, but the two have become inextricably intertwined, along with the ethical problems each raises. The fitness of a young accident victim as an organ donor might tempt a physician into sustaining his life artificially for an unduly long time until the transplant operation was set up. This has led to the suggestion in the Harvard report that the dying patient's physician work absolutely independently of the transplant team--"This is advisable in order to avoid any appearance of self-interest by the physicians involved"[35] --and to Leon Kass's admonition that decisions about when to permit a patient to die must be "based solely on a consideration of the welfare of the dying patient, rather than on a consideration of benefits that accrue to others. "[36]

A related question is how to determine the attitude of the dying patient towards the salvaging of the organs that have been a unique component of his bodily life. There are two proposals put forth. Jesse Dukeminier and David Sanders propose that organs should be routinely salvaged from dead patients, especially if they are young and fit. Every patient should be presumed to have consented to the procedure unless he or she has explicitly said something to the contrary. The surviving family has no rights of its own to deny permission. They argue that this procedure would maximize the number of organs made available, save people the bother of registering as donors or carrying special identification, and spare the doctors from having to make "ghoulish" overtones to the dying patient or to the bereaved family.[37]

Another proposal is contained in the Uniform Anatomical Gift Act (UAGA) drawn up by a special committee chaired by Professor E. Blythe Stasin. It has been adopted by virtually every state legislature in this country. It decrees that a patient would have to consent to the procedure beforehand if his or her organs were to be removed at death. Again, the next of kin could make no objections. The act is "based on the belief that each individual should be able to control the disposition of his body after death without having his wishes frustrated by anyone, including his next of kin. "[38]

Paul Ramsey supports the UAGA because it gives the chance to the donor to give himself to another, and protects the whole process from turning into a mechanical harvest of spare parts. "A society will be a better human community in which giving and receiving is the rule, not taking for the sake of good to come."[39] William May criticizes the proposal for the routine salvaging of organs because it ignores the fact of human horror over death, often expressed in the symbols of art and literature as a "devourer":

> In the course of life a breakdown in health is often accompanied by a sense that one has been exhausted and burned out by a world that has consumed all one's resources. The hospital traditionally offered a respite from a devouring world and the possibility of restoration. The healing mission of the hospital is obscured, however, if the hospital itself becomes the arch-symbol of a world that devours. Categorical salvaging of organs suggests that eventually and ultimately the process of consumption that dominates the outer world must now be consummated in the hospital. One's very vitals must be inventoried, extracted and distributed by the state on behalf of social order. What is left over is utterly unusable husk.[40]

Such an association could tend to break down the trust upon which the arts of healing depend.

Gerald Leach, on the other hand, finds the denial of rights to the surviving kin distasteful in two similar proposals being considered in Britain:

> ...Both these proposals ignore one very important factor. Although most people tell pollsters that they would like their organs used, very few can have thought deeply about what this might mean to their families. As a society we have already reduced the ritual of mourning to a psychologically dangerous minimum. How are we really going to feel when other people walk about with our dead children's or husband's or wife's living hearts?...I, for one, will never forgive the doctors involved in the first British heart transplant, who took the donor's heart before his pregnant wife knew of his death. Or the society which almost completely ignored this in the excitement of their immediate success.[41]

Modern medicine, it seems, is no more successful than traditional religion in laying to rest the fears and problems of death.

Chapter 6

Allocation of
Scarce Medical Resources

The Cases

1   Two businessmen make application for admission to their
local hospital's hemodialysis program at approximately the same
time. Both are in advanced stages of renal failure. In order to
survive, each must use kidney machines to cleanse his blood.
Unfortunately, when they apply there is only one machine available. Each session with the machine takes about twelve to
fourteen hours; two such sessions are required a week; and the
hospital already has thirteen people enrolled in their program.
The nearest hospital with a similar machine is more than two
hundred miles away.

    The doctors in charge of the program can make no distinction
between the two men on the grounds of medical suitability. Both
are in their late thirties, intelligent, otherwise in good health,
and apparently quite capable of sticking to a demanding medical
regimen. An appeal is made to the hospital ethics board for
help in the selection. The board decides to select a candidate
by flipping a coin. The two men are called in and told that the
board does not wish to choose between them on the basis of their
worth to society, to their families, or by any other value-
dependent criteria. They wish to leave the matter to fate. One
of the men protests. He argues that he would feel much more
content, even if he were rejected for the program, if some
reason could be given. Flipping a coin is much too cold and
impersonal a way to decide to save or kill a man, he says, but
adds that he would abide by such a decision if they will not
change their minds. The board asks the other man what he
thinks. He says he is content to let the coin decide. "I'd rather
not win just because I was thought to be a 'better citizen.' I'd

never be able to live up to it. " One of the board members flips a coin. The man who protested wins the toss. He goes on the program.

2   A small-town government receives some revenue-sharing funds from the federal government that it decides to earmark for medical programs. The town council members discuss how it should be spent. One member points out that in the rural schools around the town almost half the children haven't been innoculated with polio vaccine. She suggests that the money purchase enough oral vaccine to treat all the school children. Another member points out that polio has almost disappeared in the last few years; and that even in the worst epidemic years only a small number of children were affected, and hardly any in their area. He recounts how his brother recently died because the town hospital didn't have enough space in its hemodialysis program. About one person a year is turned away to die, he says. Here is a more immediate need, he concludes. The council votes to contribute their money to the local hospital for the purchase of a dialysis machine.

3   An election replaces all the members of a rural county government with members of another party. An analysis is made of how the government's budget is structured, and it is discovered that almost all the county's medical budget is contributed to the nearest hospital in the county's largest town, to be used as the hospital directors see fit. They discover further that most of the money goes to augment the salaries of the physicians at the hospital. "We've got to pay more to hold doctors in remote areas like this, " a spokesman for the hospital explains. The new county government decides to cancel contributions to the hospital. They inform each taxpayer in the county that the money is going to purchase basic medical programs according to their wishes. They can indicate their choices among comprehensive programs of either innoculation, water floridation, or basic dental care. The taxpayers, most of them farmers, are enthusiastic about the plan. They support the county government against the protests of the local hospital board. During the following year a comprehensive program of innoculation against basic diseases is administered through county extension offices, and about a fourth of the hospital staff,

their salaries reduced, leave the town for other jobs. Some re-
sign in protest over governmental interference with medicine.
Many of the hospital's more sophisticated services, such as
major surgery, long-term intensive care, and some research
programs, are discontinued because of lack of personnel.

The Issues

Health needs are limitless--everybody saved from a deadly
infection by an antibiotic lives to be vulnerable to accidents or
chronic sickness or the diseases of old age--while medical
resources are limited. Every dollar given to purchase military
armaments or a city park could have been spent on a public
health clinic. Every dollar a citizen gives in taxes he or she
could have used to purchase more sophisticated medical treatment at home.

Two obvious questions arise from the discrepancy between
limitless needs and limited means. One is how are we to decide who gets what is available when there isn't enough to go
around? Are only the rich to be healthy? Even if they are,
what if two of them compete for the same scarce life-saving
medical resource, for example, a dialysis machine? The recently published Burton Report estimated that it would cost
$701 million to buy and maintain enough machines to service
the fifty thousand patients who develop endstage kidney disease
each year in this country. It would cost $1.043 billion by the
fifth year of the program, between $1.816 and $2.702 billion
by the fifteenth. The report recommended that the number of
patients be winnowed to six to eight thousand a year (selecting
the most ideal patients) to make the programs more economic-
ally feasible. The solution to the problem of how to select
these patients could be used to allocate heart-lung machines,
organs available for transplants, innoculations, dental care,
and all other scarce resources.

Another question, perhaps a more basic one, is what should
be made available in the first place? How much should a
society spend on medicine? How big a piece of the pie should
be cut for building dialysis machines, funding cancer research,
or immunizing a whole population against preventable diseases
like measles and polio? In this chapter, we consider responses
to each question in turn.

Allocation of Scarce Supplies

Writers have suggested three ways to allocate scarce available medical resources among the needy--for example, a kidney donated by a dying patient: select patients for care according to their relative worth, select them blindly by lottery, or select no one at all and let everyone suffer. Edmond Cahn finds the idea of using a lottery to decide human life so repugnant that he argues if not all can be saved than none should be saved. A crisis in human lives "involves stakes too high for gambling and responsibilities too deep for destiny, " he says while discussing the legal case often cited as having the most implications for this problem of medical ethics (although the circumstances were quite different). In United States v. Holmes, the defendant, a ship's mate in charge of a lifeboat after his ship had sunk, was charged with manslaughter for his decision to throw overboard fourteen male passengers to lighten the boat. The judge, in charging the jury, said that if the sailors on the lifeboat had been indispensable for navigation, then the victims to be sacrificed among the passengers should have been chosen by lot so that there would have been no covert discrimination among them. Human beings have equal worth when any must be selected for doom. According to Cahn, the situation in the lifeboat or in a hospital short of medical resources requires that individual human beings declare themselves willing to sacrifice themselves. If insufficient numbers of free volunteers come forth, then the community which fails to produce its own heroes condemns itself to an equal death for all.[1]

Leo Shatin, on the other hand, thinks that a community could make decisions less drastically. He reasons that as there is no way to escape making value judgments about who is more deserving in a crisis situation; the criteria to be applied in selection should at least be made explicit and open to argument and adjustment. Polls of public opinion could establish criteria according to profession (clergy rated higher than businessmen, for example) and according to functions in the community (mothers rated higher than spinsters). He rejects the notion of a process of random selection because it would often reward "socially disvalued qualities by giving their bearers the same medical care

opportunities as those received by the bearers of socially valued
qualities. "[2]

Using Social Worth for Patient Selection

In 1961, Dr. Belding H. Scribner set up a program guided
by principles similar to those Shatin has in mind in order to
screen patients at the Swedish Hospital in Seattle, Washington,
for hemodialysis treatment. The Admissions and Policies
Committee of the Seattle Artificial Kidney Center at Swedish
Hospital was comprised of a lawyer, a clergyman, a housewife,
a banker, a labor leader, and two physicians, all of whom remained anonymous to the public, the patients, and the members
of the hospital staff. They were commissioned to set their own
guidelines and to apply them. The only advice physicians gave
them was to reject automatically children who hadn't reached
puberty (treatment slows or prevents puberty because children
often don't have the stamina for the treatment regimen) or adults
over forty-five (whose bodies are more prone to develop serious
complications).

The committee decided to base its decisions on criteria of
social worth. Patients were accepted or rejected on the basis
of how much education they had, how easy it would be for their
spouses to remarry, how active they were in church work.
Although both the patients and the committee approved of the
committee's work, both groups agonized over the procedure.
A patient who was chosen to live said, "What a dreadful decision!
It's like trying to play God. Frankly, I'm surprised the doctors
were able to round up seven people who were willing to take the
job. " The banker on the committee said, "I've never had any
idea how a kidney works, and I still don't. But I do have reservations about the moral aspects of the propriety of choosing A
and not B, for whatever reason. I have often asked myself, as
a human being, do I have that right? I don't really think I do.
I finally came to the conclusion that we are not making a moral
choice here. We are picking guinea pigs for experimental purposes. This happens to be true; it also happens to be the way I
rationalize my presence on this committee. " One of the physicians said, "Being a medical man, I sometimes hear it via the
grapevine when a patient whom we have passed over dies. Each

time this happens there always comes a feeling of deep regret--
perhaps we chose the wrong man. One can just never face these
situations without feeling a little sick inside. "[3]

The author of the article from which these quotations were
taken felt uncomfortable not so much with the fact that decisions
had to be made as with the criteria for selection. "On the basis
of the past year's record, a candidate who plans to come before
this committee would seem well-advised to father a great many
children, then to throw away all his money, and finally to fall
ill in a season when there will be a minimum of competition
from other men dying of the same disease. " David Sanders and
Jesse Dukeminier who studied the committee's work were more
explicit in their criticism of a procedure that turned middle-class
values into criteria for deciding who would live. They find "a
disturbing picture of the bourgeoisie sparing the bourgeoisie....
The Pacific Northwest is not the place for a Henry David Thoreau
with bad kidneys. "[4]

Using a Lottery for Patient Selection

The Holmes case and the Seattle committee loom large in
the thinking of other writers who favor a lottery for its random
disregard of volatile moral evaluations. "Randomness as a
moral principle" writes Paul Freund, "deserves serious study. "[5]
Paul Ramsey points up a disturbing logical consequence to
selecting patients on the basis of their social worth. What if a
patient's morals degenerate and he or she starts to carouse and
run around or gets divorced while on dialysis; should such a
patient be dropped from the program so that a position could be
offered to someone else more sober? [6] For the same reasons
that Sanders and Dukeminier state, he feels uncomfortable with
the use of middle-class standards for judging a person worthy
to live. He also concurs with another argument in their study
that shifting the onus of evaluation to a physician or a psychiatrist would simply be shifting the same kind of criteria into
other hands. Medical suitability is often "doctored" to suit a
person's social worth. He also rejects as too severe Cahn's
argument that if no one volunteers to sacrifice himself, all
should die.

Ramsey favors using a lottery. Its use acknowledges each patient's equal right to treatment and gives each an equal opportunity to get it. He suggests that the process have three stages: First, rules could be announced in advance which are not discriminatory, but based on statistical medical probabilities. Children under the age of puberty and adults over forty-five are bad risks for dialysis. Secondly, dialysis machines could be assigned on a first-come, first-served basis. The applicant with the most seniority whose health was still unimpaired enough for treatment would automatically be granted a place on a suddenly vacant machine. Third, lots could be cast. All three methods could be used separately or in sequence until selection was made. He concludes:

> The immediate translation of a covenant of righteousness and
> faithfulness among men cannot be either that all must wait and
> die or be rescued together or that some are to be saved accord-
> ing to inequalities of their social worth. Instead, the translation
> of fidelity among men must surely be into the principle that
> every person in the longboat of hospital practice has equal worth
> as a human being. When these worths are in competition for
> sparse medical resources, when not everyone can be saved who
> needs a particular life-saving remedy, random patient selection
> would seem to be the only way to acknowledge and adhere to the
> inherent worth every man has as a man among men. [7]

Ramsey adopts one qualification to this process from Paul Freund: When a group of human beings are reduced to needing "focused criteria" to survive, they can choose among themselves according to their immediate social value. Freund cites the decision made in North Africa in World War II to use scarce supplies of penicillin to cure syphilis rather than serious war wounds. The men wounded in brothels could be more quickly returned to the front than those wounded in battle. [8]

A similar exception could be made when a disaster such as an earthquake or an aerial bomb strikes a large population at once and wounds far more people than there are medical supplies to treat, creating a need for a system of triage. The survivors are divided into three groups. Those seriously wounded with little hope of recovery receive no treatment; hopeless cases, they are left to die without being allowed to consume any precious resources. Those only slightly injured who can function without medication also receive no treatment. They are assumed able to help in attending to the third or middle group: wounded persons who, if treated, could recover sufficiently to help in the rescue and rebuilding operations. Perhaps even slightly wounded physicians would be treated if this enabled them to better serve the whole group.

Systematic Selection

James F. Childress, after reviewing most of the literature mentioned here, chooses a more systematic procedure of random selection. First, the patient group should be screened objectively by doctors using medical criteria, automatically rejecting people not acceptable for reasons of age or their suffering from other diseases. These criteria should be broad lest there develop a process of "fine comparison" at this stage-- rejecting one patient because he is slightly older or slightly less healthy looking than another. If after this selection there are still more applicants than resources, a lottery should choose among them. This process is a fair way, Childress thinks, for granting equal rights to all human beings in the face of inadequate medical supplies and the limited capacity of individual human beings for altruism.[9]

Frederic B. Westervelt, Jr., M.D., replies to Childress and through him to Ramsey and Freund by criticizing the lottery method. He argues that it operates under false pretenses in that it does not really disregard patients' social worth. Primarily upper- and middle-class people are fortunate enough to enjoy early diagnosis of their ills. Consequently, he reasons, only they get a shot at scarce resources. Discrimination has already occurred in pre-selection. From another tack, Westervelt asks what if a doctor decides that a patient with an ailing kidney could be treated with drugs and diet for a long time before any need for dialysis arose. Would this patient lose his or her place in the "first-come, first-served" line when dialysis became necessary just because some less-scarce remedy worked for a time? What if a patient selected by a lottery was cantankerous and would not get along well with the doctors or lived too far from the dialysis center to be able to meet regular appointments? Should patients

such as these be replaced by more polite, more reasonable, or
more accessible patients?

Westervelt finally argues that a system of triage should be
applied by a physician who takes into account the patient's morale,
health, and convenience, as well as his or her social worth.
Someone should be willing to take the moral responsibility for
the decision:

> Triage should remain the purview of those answerable for the
> program, who must avail themselves of all relevant sources of
> information, opinion, and guidance. The key to responsible
> action lies with the responsible physician. So long as his de-
> cisions, however effected, are forthright, conscionable, subject
> to discussion and consonant with his obligation to individual and
> group, these difficulties can be met. If otherwise, far more is
> in jeopardy than the patient with failing kidneys.[10]

Choosing Among Medical Programs

Some writers who take up the second question of what medical
resources should be made available in the first place throw up
their hands in despair. Ramsey writes that "...the question of
setting priorities, which--tragically, perhaps--must be faced
and thought through by the medical profession and by society in
general...is a question that is almost if not altogether incorri-
gible to rational determination."[11]   Leach writes:

> The trouble here is that there is absolutely no logical way of
> choosing except by some measurable quality like benefit-cost
> ratios. One cannot make intuitive judgments that it is better or
> worse to spend X on prolonging one life for a year than to spend
> it, say, on alleviating the misery of arthritis in fifty people.
> Yet though medicine has traditionally put its greatest efforts into
> life-prolonging, what...benefit-cost figures show is that for the
> health and wealth of society less dramatic goals can often be a
> relatively far better bargain.[12]

After an extensive review of the literature on the subject, Henry
Beecher writes: "It was a considerable disappointment to the
writer, after the examination of more than a dozen areas where
scarce resources were involved, to find statements of only the
most rudimentary principles of procedure."[13]

Beecher's study of the manifold causes of scarcity emphasizes the dilemma. He begins with a history of the development of certain medical techniques such as anesthesia, insulin, penicillin and the Chamberlen forceps for aiding difficult child delivery. All were scarce at the beginning because they were untested and not yet widely reproduced, but they stayed scarce for different lengths of time for very different reasons. The Chamberlen family kept their discovery secret for many years in order to sell it privately for high prices. It could have been easily imitated and widely distributed. William Thomas Green Morton kept secret the active agents of his "Lethon" used as an anesthesia because he felt careful experimentation was necessary before its use became widespread. Public pressure finally forced him to reveal the components and to distribute the resource. Penicillin was initially a scarce resource because it could not be produced fast enough to meet the many demands for it. The use of insulin developed slowly as it was experimentally given only to severe cases until the proper dosages and the possible side effects were determined. Avarice, rudimentary production, or caution can cause scarcity.

Other kinds of human attitudes also play a part. In certain states there is a prejudice against using "racially mixed" blood. All fresh blood and blood plasma must be designated according to the race of its donor so that a squeamish patient might refuse it. This could radically restrict the amount of blood available to a particular patient at a certain time. Jehovah's Witnesses voluntarily limit the medical resources available to them when they refuse all blood transfusions on religious principles. American Navy men in the eighteenth and nineteenth centuries suffered from scurvy because of their ignorance of or prejudice against the successful British practice of putting limes in the diet of British Navy men as a prophylactic. There are finally ethical restraints against using certain resources which, as a result, become scarce. The Uniform Anatomical Gift Act stipulates that only donor-volunteered organs can be used in transplant surgery. Similar restraints against experimentation with children, prisoners, or unconsenting human subjects likewise retard the development of medical technology.

Finally, Beecher points to the inertia of medical research itself. Christiaan Barnard's spectacular early success with

heart transplants attracted to his transplant research a lot of
money which thereby became less available for other medical
programs. Cancer research likewise absorbs the money that
could be used to inoculate children in rural areas or in Third
World countries against measles, polio, and other controllable
diseases. Politics plays a role as well. Well-to-do white
people are perhaps more interested in the diseases that threaten
them such as cancer and, consequently, support research in
these areas more strongly. Sickle-cell anemia research and
treatment began to advance much more rapidly after black
political groups began to publicize their problems and solicit
support.

When Ramsey purviews the politics of medical distribution,
he finds himself perplexed and loath to make any principled decision to favor one kind of medicine over another: "A civilization consists of many different qualities and levels of activities
as does medical practice. In the recovery of Europe after World
War II, opera houses were rebuilt along with housing for the
homeless."[14]

Leach draws out several hidden paradoxes in the muddle.
Mass prevention campaigns against infectious diseases usually
wind up increasing medical costs. Prevention costs more than
the treatment of the few who used to get the disease. Likewise
"the cost of screening everybody could still be much higher than
the conventional approach of letting these diseases take hold
and trying to cure the few advanced cases that one can."[15] As
great numbers of the population become immune to curable
diseases, their medical needs rise in sophistication. Soon
everyone who survives polio, the measles, diabetes, and so
forth, will be threatened only by cancer and beyond that death
itself. The principle at work here is that as "the standards of
what it means to be 'healthy' rise...the total of reported illness
actually rises."[16] Those who finally reach this plateau will
probably be grateful if, while they were being innoculated, sophisticated research against the disease that now threatens
them was being carried on continuously.

If one follows the reasoning of Ramsey and Leach there would
seem to be no way out of the dilemma of inequitable distribution.
There is no way to weigh conflicting needs against each other,
and even if there were, one need would eventually replace the

other. Perhaps there is a certain amount of comfort that can be taken from all this. Perhaps something like Adam Smith's "invisible hand" directing the economic market directs the medical market as well. Perhaps society as a whole is making decisions about the advancement of medicine or the distribution of resources through a process of balancing conflicting interests. On this level the process is immune to meddling or resistent to programming, depending on your point of view; no "system" would distribute goods any better than the current free market does. One could take comfort in hoping that the society is serving its own best interests far better than any direct political control of the process could. Laissez-faire could be letting a fundamentally benign process go its cautious, merry way.

Organized Allocation

Recent studies suggest that mere patchwork efforts simply do not cure the ills of poverty. Paul Starr discovers that since the institution of Medicaid in the United States in 1964, poor people actually visit physicians more frequently than those who are not poor. The overall average number of visits a year for the poor in 1964 was 4.3; for the not poor, 4.6. By 1973, the frequency was 5.6 compared to 4.9, although the children and elderly of the poor still go less often than those of the not poor. The same studies from which he draws his data suggest why the poor see doctors more often: the poor are sicker. "The prevalence rates per 1,000 persons for arthritis are 297.8 in low-income families versus 159.8 in upper-income families; for diabetes, 74.1 versus 30.5; for heart conditions, 139.3 versus 66.6; for hypertension, 172.7 versus 105.3; for impairments of the back and spine, 102.8 versus 52.2."[17]

A study of mortality rates among white males between the ages of twenty-five and sixty-four suggests as well that health is more a function of income and education than the availability of medical care in itself. Evelyn M. Kitagawa and Philip M. Hauser found that in 1960, deaths in this group were 80 percent higher for men in families earning less than $2,000 than for men in families earning over $10,000. Men of the same age with fewer than five years of schooling had a mortality rate 64 percent higher than male college graduates.[18]

One response to these facts could be that making people healthy
is not primarily the responsibility of the medical profession, or
a function of allocating medical attention more equitably, but
requires a vast political and economic reordering of the whole
society. It lies, in any case, outside the province of medical
ethics as such. Starr reviews in his article the recent literature following a related tack. What he calls the "politics of
therapeutic nihilism" tries to strip away the false illusions of
medical promise. Ivan Illich, a most eloquent nihilist of this
sort, argues in his Medical Nemesis that advances in health and
life expectancy grow from improvements in the standard of
living, and from relatively simple medical technology such as
immunization. He thinks a dangerous tendency has been growing to put misplaced trust in antibiotics, psychoactive drugs,
and medications, and at the same time to consider more and
more of the normal vicissitudes of human life as sickness needing medical relief. Furthermore, doctors and medicine, as the
burgeoning of malpractice litigation suggests, have been likely
to hurt as much as to help human life. He concludes bluntly,
"less access to the present health system would, contrary to
political rhetoric, benefit the poor."[19]
Starr himself hopes the current criticism might prick the
modern medical establishment into becoming more responsible
for the health of the whole society it serves. He concedes the
points to Illich and others writing in this vein that "environment
and behavior are principle determinants of health and life expectancy; medical care plays a relatively small part.... If one
wishes to equalize health, equalizing medical care is probably
not the most effective strategy." He agrees that some means
must be found to put limits on the expense of medicine, but he
also believes:

> ...the expansion and improvement of medical services probably
> have had a positive effect on health. The reduction of risks at
> the margin has enhanced personal security. Had it not been for
> medical care, mortality rates might be higher. Medicine has
> useful functions other than saving lives, such as relieving dis-
> comfort and disability and making sickness more bearable for
> patients and their families. Further investments in certain
> areas of medical care, such as maternal and child health, may
> continue to yield positive returns.... The hard and discriminat-

ing eye that distinguishes useless from effective practices in
medicine, or other fields, need not be unfriendly to the concern
for equality. To improve the effectiveness of social services,
we will have to be especially attentive to inequalities. It makes
no sense to add more where there is already too much. [20]

In an earlier article, Starr casts a sympathetic eye on comprehensive new programs for genuinely equitable allocation of
medical resources, such as the one David Rutstein outlines in
his Blueprint for Medical Care. [21]

Comprehensive Health Plans

David Rutstein's blueprint calls for putting physicians on
salary and eliminating solo practice. The Department of Health,
Education, and Welfare would control all medical services from
emergency treatment to preventive medicine, dispensing authority through regional directorships. Each directorship would
control emergency centers with centralized communications
and transportation, neighborhood reception centers for minor
medical problems, community hospitals for inpatient care, and
researching-teaching hospitals for special cases and carefully
controlled experimentation. The reception centers would also
serve as referral points for more complex problems, and as
bases for home-visiting services. The community hospitals
would house the offices of general practitioners. Rural regions
would be affiliated with urban centers to assure the equal distribution of personnel and resources to all sections of the society. The Federal Health Board (modeled after the Federal
Reserve Board) would maintain a quality-control system over
the programs and personnel.

Rutstein would also systematize the education of medical
personnel. Trained paraprofessionals would relieve physicians
of all ordinary and routine treatment and care. General practitioners would be paid as much as specialists to attract young
doctors into general practice.

Possibly the most characteristic aspect of Rutstein's plan is
a proposal to put all aspects of the program under the review of
two different kinds of control systems to collect and analyze
and to feed back data on the quality of care:

... a guidance system to measure, follow, and interpret ac-
complishments and failures, and to lay out a course for future
programs; and an early warning system to identify sudden out-
croppings of undesirable health events that may demand immediate action. Both systems will be focused on the occurrence of
unnecessary disease, disability, and untimely death and negative indices of the quality of care. The guidance system will
determine and compare their statistical distribution throughout
the country and in each medical care region, while the early
warning system will signal and evaluate the epidemiological
occurrence of individual sentinel health events.[22]

Instead of an invisible hand, there would be a continuously rov-
ing, all-seeing computerized eye looking into all aspects of the
country's health needs, seeing to it that all preventable health
problems would be prevented, and that research money was
allocated in precise proportion to the needs.

Paul Starr criticizes Rutstein's system for its rigidity on its
lowest levels:

The chief defect of the "blueprint," as I see it, lies in neither
its putative technocratic nor its utopian aspects, but rather in
the basic postulate of a single and unified system. The danger
in such a plan is that it creates a network of local monopolies;
each district has one institutional system available for health
care. For water supply that is convenient and logical; for medical purposes, it is not. Rutstein's argument for constructing
such a system is that it would be more efficient because it
eliminates duplication, permits long-run planning and budgeting,
and cuts administrative cost. All of these may be true, but
the system would nonetheless provide limited alternatives for
those who become dissatisfied with the care they receive. In
favoring short-run considerations of efficiency, Rutstein has
sacrificed non-economic considerations of choice. Furthermore,
by protecting local systems against competition, he may in the
long run have sacrificed efficiency as well, since it may be
possible for very inefficient local programs to continue without challenge.[23]

Starr suggests finding a place in a system like Rutstein's
for a voucher system. The government would permit its citizens to opt for membership in the "health maintenance organization" that best suited them. In these organizations, health
care from treating the simplest infection to the most elaborate

brain surgery is made available to its members who pay a flat fee every month. The money goes for hiring doctors, purchasing medical facilities, and perhaps renting special supplies and facilities when the rare occasion calls for them. Each particular organization would reflect the needs of its particular members. Perhaps one might hire a plastic surgeon, another, an extra general practitioner. Each organization would compete with others for patients and doctors. The government could contribute a certain percentage of each individual member's fee. Something like Rutstein's Federal Health Board could regulate the salaries of doctors in each organization, standardize costs, distribute health resources to various parts of the country, and fund research.

Starr thinks there is a need for a diversified program such as his modification of Rutstein's to replace the disorganization in health care which now goes by the false name of pluralism: "Entrepreneur professional practice, hospital empires, incomplete and complicated insurance coverage, categorical federal benefits, and projects, overlapping federal, state and local programs, unintegrated public health services and disjointed emergency measures--serve none of us well. What I am proposing here is an organized system that uses competition in a premeditated fashion: competition under constraint. "[24]

If systems such as Rutstein and Starr's wouldn't solve the problems of how to distribute scarce resources, they could at least make the distribution process public and open to critical review. The whole society might be able to take a more conscious, active role in determining how their health needs are met, the poor in health and pocketbook included.

Chapter 7

The Eugenic Medicine of the Future Through In Vitro Fertilization, Genetic Surgery, and Cloning

The Cases

1   A scientist working in conjunction with a urologist in private practice perfects the technique of in vitro fertilization. Five patients of the urologist suffer from a defect in their reproductive organs; their Fallopian tubes are blocked; sperm cannot reach their ova for fertilization. With the new technique ova from each woman are removed from their ovaries and fertilized by their spouses' sperm in test tubes. The resulting zygotes are cultivated until they have grown to several thousand cells, at which point they are implanted into the uterus of each woman. Continual monitoring of their pregnancies indicate that all but one of the women are bearing normal fetuses. The defective fetus is aborted. The other four women give birth to normal babies. All the women are enjoined to secrecy about the experiment, lest, the scientist explains, there be a public outcry against his experiments before they are perfected.

2   Geneticists working with fruit flies have developed a technique of genetic manipulation called "transformation." In this procedure, genetic material from one type of fly can be used to direct a specific genetic change in a second type of fly. Embryos from one Drosophilia strain are treated with DNA from flies of another strain. In a small percentage of the cases genetic mosaics resulted--flies with genetic characteristics of both strains distributed randomly throughout their bodies. The geneticists can find no way to predict how or when this distribution will occur.

Bacterial geneticists have developed techniques of genetic manipulation called "transduction." In this procedure genes are transferred from one bacteria to another by a virus. In one of their experiments, a gene-controlling production of arginase (a blood serum enzyme essential for the proper metabolism of the amino acid arginine) has been transferred from a rabbit to a rat by a virus.

A team of scientists intrigued by these experiments apply for a grant to study the possibilities of developing these techniques into surgical procedures for the treatment of genetic diseases in humans. They recognize that the obstacles are formidable. Even if a gene could be isolated for transfer, it would be extremely difficult to direct it precisely to the target tissue. If misdirected it might effect the whole organism randomly and with possible monstrous results (defective fruit flies can be dispensed with more easily than defective human fetuses). Then, assuming that the targeting was precise and that a specific genetic disorder could be eliminated, it is quite likely that the genotype of the treated individuals would remain basically unchanged so that they could pass on defective genes to some of their children, who would also require genetic surgery of the same type. They reason that the possible medical advances are worth the risks. Their project is funded. They begin to work with human cell cultures.

3   Scientists have been able to reproduce frogs by cloning, a form of asexual reproduction similar to reproducing plants from cuttings. The nucleus of the egg of a female frog is cut out and replaced by a nucleus obtained from a body cell of another frog (or the same frog). Because each cell contains the code for the entire genetic makeup of its parent body, the resulting embryo grows to become an identical twin of the frog which yielded the body cells, without the random mixing of genetic characteristics that occurs in normal fertilization. If the cells are taken from the mother frog, she produces a twin of herself.

A researcher begins experiments to reproduce mice by the same process. She has in mind the eventual development of a technique allowing human females to reproduce themselves by the implantation of the nucleus of a mother's cell into her own ovum. A radical feminist, she hopes to make it possible for women to produce children if they wish without male intervention. The technique could also be used to permit parents to have children if the father were sterile.   Each person in the couple could be cloned.

The Issues

Looking to the future is looking beyond medicine as curing or even preventing disease to its becoming a science of creating human beings who are immune to diseases and perhaps eventually immune to aging and dying.   Three experiments in this direction--in vitro fertilization, genetic surgery, and cloning-- are already in initial stages at work with insects, frogs, and mammals, and perhaps with cultures of human cells.   The question they raise for medical ethics is simply whether their technologies should be restricted to helping sterile couples procreate or to curing certain genetic diseases, or should be allowed to develop into a eugenic program to improve the "breed" of human beings.

It is a hard question to keep focused as research into the intricacies of DNA probes the structure underlying all forms of organic life--in plants, animals, viruses, and integral human beings; manipulative genetic techniques would have myriad uses outside medicine.   Cloning could revolutionize animal breeding. One prize cow or bull or sheep or pig could be reproduced over and over again without gambling on recessive gene appearance. Genetic engineering could order a desired change in a particular animal to make it more resistant to a prevalent disease or to adapt it to a harsh climate.   Transferring the appropriate enzyme set to wheat, maize, rice, and beets would substantially reduce the need for artificial nitrogenous fertilizers and increase the protein yield. [1] Similar techniques could revolutionize childbearing.   Individual couples sterile for one reason or another could have a natural child cloned for themselves.   Genetic surgery could correct the faulty metabolism of genetically defective fetuses.   Perhaps eventually genes could be doctored to produce immunization against all the debilitating diseases a person would ever face in a lifetime.   Diabetics would be freed of ever needing to take another shot of insulin, the blind be made to see, the deaf hear; the possibilities seem endless.

Consequently some writers grow uneasy about where genetic manipulation would stop.   They single out an important portion of the new biology to question whether the process of engineering cures should expand into a process of engineering whole new forms of human life. When in vitro fertilization becomes possible, a fetus could be conceived outside its natural mother's womb with the sperm of a donor and then implanted into the womb of a woman willing to rent space for nine months. It might then be a short step to developing even more exquisite techniques such as gestating the fetus for the full nine months under glass, monitoring its every movement, and "correcting" any undesirable traits or incorporating desirable traits through genetic engineering. From these advances it might later be possible to propagate animal-human hybrids, such as intelligent, armed porpoises for underwater work, bio-machines (cyborgs) for menial labor, and specially engineered humans for special purposes: legless astronauts, huge-lunged scuba divers, very narrow chimney sweeps.

For Paul Ramsey, such an extension would be tantamount to human beings committing "species suicide." Now humans are shaped by a weaving together of their own efforts to direct their lives and the unforeseeable twistings of fate; with their own biology completely in their own hands they would become demi-gods, as different from human beings as they now are from their primate ancestors.

For Harold Green, another writer considered in this chapter, the decision must be made now whether the expansion would be allowed. Even if the techniques are not now sophisticated they soon will be if research with them continues, and then, he feels certain, it will be impossible to monitor or restrict their use. Irresponsible nations or Dr. Frankensteins will unleash a new type of life upon an already overburdened earth. To prevent this from happening, perhaps the acknowledged goods of their restricted use might have to be sacrificed.

A retort to Green's argument could be that all technologies bring promise and danger--nuclear fission, for example. Willard Gaylin, in writing about some dangers of genetic screening, says: "It is important that the new spirit of self-criticism not condemn legitimate pursuits by confusing them with questionable applications. Anti-technology with its implicit self-hatred is often a product of careless thinking in an unfamiliar area."[2] Comfort could come from realizing that many eugenic techniques avail-

able today--such as enforced selective breeding and euthanasia--
remain unused even by existing totalitarian regimes.[3] Finally,
one could point to the heartening example set by the genetic
scientists recently meeting at the Asilomar Conference in Cali-
fornia who decided voluntarily to police their own dangerous experiments with fabricating artificial viruses (recombining DNA).
It was, one commentator remarked, a "rare if not unique example of safety precautions being imposed on a technical development before instead of after the first occurrence of the hazard."[4]

But these words and examples do not completely lay the specter
of modern biological eugenics to rest. Genetically engineering
a whole new genotype would be more than applying another technology; it would mean the dawning of a whole new age of human
production, perhaps entailing irrevocable loss if, as some scientists suspect, many cloned or engineered humans would be
sterile and unable to reproduce in any other way. The scientists at Asilomar made a reasoned decision not to take certain
risks to achieve certain scientific goals because the risks were
too great. However, certain other scientists considered in previous chapters such as Delgado and Skinner, and others considered in this chapter such as Lederberg, Muller, and the
philosopher Joseph Fletcher make it clear that they consider
human fabrication not so much a risk as an enterprise of greatly
exciting promise. By the time similarly thinking scientists
were ready to clone a man, their demands or persuasions
might prove irresistible to those of Ramsey and Green.

The discussion in this chapter focuses on the eugenic application of the new biology--the particular concern of medical ethics.
For context it begins with a look at several past traditions of
eugenics which have already held out the promise of making more
"perfect" human beings.

Eugenics

The motives for programs of eugenics have varied considerably. Sir Francis Galton, the father of modern eugenics, wrote
in the late nineteenth century that a human being needs physique,
ability, and character to be a fit human being. The foundation
for these traits he believed to be an inheritable genetic sub-
structure of suitable genes. When biologists learned enough

about genes, humans could begin to breed themselves as they had learned to breed prize animals. People with good traits could be encouraged to breed with each other; people with bad traits not to. Under the influence of his thinking many states in the early twentieth century enacted laws forbidding marriage by criminals, imbeciles, alcoholics, the feebleminded, and the insane. Not many are still on the books, but there are still restrictions against marriage between people with venereal diseases.[5] To "purify" their breeding stock, the Nazis experimented with negative eugenics by trying to exterminate what they thought were inferior races, and with positive eugenics by encouraging the mating of bona fide Aryan couples. Today scientists would revive Galton's goals with new methods for new reasons. Some people argue that the human race is suffering a gradual decline in its genetic health that only scientific eugenics could reverse.

To understand the modern concern, we need a sense of how modern medicine is affecting the human gene pool. The total number of genetic defects an individual or a population carries is called its genetic load. Most such defects go unnoticed. Many genetically defective fetuses miscarry, and the more serious birth defects are often quickly fatal. Many mutations go unnoticed in children and adults because they are only slightly expressed, slightly harmful, or recessive. Although everybody inherits recessive genes from one parent and corresponding normal genes from another and are thus heterozygous for that gene, only rarely do two detrimental recessive genes line up making a person homozygous for that gene. Only then are any overtly harmful effects of recessive genes expressed; even then, the expression is usually only momentary, either because it is fatal, or because unhindered natural selection works against the build-up of mutations in the human gene pool by discriminating against the persons who would reproduce them. Very often homozygotes, if they survive infancy, don't live until the age of reproduction; and often their births frighten their parents into not producing any more children and thereby into restricting even further the number of heterozygote persons. In the modern age, however, modern medicine hinders natural selection with increasing success. People suffering from diabetes, phenylketonuria, and other diseases can now live healthy productive and reproductive lives. Every diabetic who lives to produce more dia-

betics increases the percentage of the population so afflicted.
In addition, modern culture has increased the use of mutagenic
agents such as X-rays, chemicals, and drugs. It is therefore
not hard to envision a point sometime in the future at which, as
H. J. Muller says, "the job of ministering to infirmities would
come to consume all the energy that society could muster for it,
leaving no surplus for general, cultural purposes."[6] In another
place, Muller writes:

> Our descendants' natural biological organization would in fact
> have disintegrated and have been replaced by complete dis-
> order. Their only connection with mankind would then be the
> historical one that we ourselves had after all been their ances-
> tors and sponsors, and the fact that their once-human material
> was still used for the purpose of converting it, artificially, in-
> to some semblance of man. However, it would in the end be far
> easier and more sensible to manufacture a complete man de
> novo, out of appropriately chosen raw materials, than to try to
> refashion into human form those pitiful relics which remained.
> For all of them would present a whole series of most intricate
> research problems, before the treatments suitable for its own
> unique set of vagaries could be decided upon.[7]

To prevent this, Muller envisions a program of positive
eugenics through voluntary use of Artificial Insemination by
Donor (A.I.D.). Particularly sound genotypes of various kinds
would donate their sperm to frozen sperm banks. Their genetic characteristics would be advertised and made available to
couples willing to reproduce proven genetic structures rather
than their own genetic load. He thinks coercion would be unnecessary because enough couples would be intelligent enough
to recognize how superior the new method would be over the
old.

> It is preposterous to suppose that, in the foreseeable future,
> knowledge would be precise enough to enable us to say what
> substitution to make in order to effect a given, desired pheno-
> typic alteration. ... But to suppose that, after it had become
> possible, men would still be bound by the reproductive tradi-
> tions of today, preferring this ultra-sophisticated method of
> improvement to the readily available one of selecting donor
> material free from the given defect of already possessing the
> desired innovation--that would be a calumny on the rationality

of the human race. It would be like supposing that in some
technically advanced society elaborate superhighways were
constructed to carry vehicles on enormous detours to avoid de-
filing hallowed domains reserved in perpetuity for their millions
of sacred cows.[8]

Joshua Lederberg, a geneticist like Muller, is not so san-
guine about the success of a voluntary positive eugenics program for these reasons: People would be likely to resist the
suppression of their diversity or individual self-expression
through their natural children; there is the danger that the
"ideal" genotypes might soon be adopted as imperative standards
with totalitarian decisions being made; even if there were sufficient volunteers, deleterious genes would continue to surface,
since most are maintained by heterozygous persons ("If we attack the heterozygotes as well as the overtly afflicted homozygotes, almost no human being will qualify"); it is not known how
long sperm can stay frozen without suffering damage; and finally, if any improvement were possible with either positive
or negative eugenics, it would happen over a long period of time
so that miscalculation wouldn't be manifest for twenty years or
more. He argues that a more "effective slogan on which to
focus as an alternative to eugenics is 'euphenics,' which means
all the alleviation of genotypic maladjustment that could be
brought about by treatment of the affected individual more ef-
ficaciously, earlier in his development. "[9]

Euphenics

Euphenics uses two types of treatment--genetic surgery and
cloning. The first is probably going to remain unfeasible for
a long time, Lederberg says. It is almost beyond reason to
expect that techniques are ever going to be perfected that would
precisely correct the genetic defects in every afflicted human
cell without disastrous side effects; and in addition, the genetic
defect that might be corrected in an individual would still be
passed on through sperm or ova to the next generation. Cloning
is more feasible, safer, and more immediately gratifying.
"Unlike other techniques of biological engineering, there might
be little delay between demonstration and use. ... If a superior

individual--and presumably, the genotype--is identified, why
not copy it directly, rather than suffer all the risks, including
those of sex determination, involved in the disruptions of
recombination. "[10]   Another advantage of clones is that their
parts are interchangeable. An organ from one could be transplanted into the body of another with no immunological rejection.
To develop this technique he suggests scientists experiment
with cloning animal-human hybrids until the process is safe
enough to be utterly predictable on real human beings. They can
be distinguished from hybrids when they "look enough like men
to grip their consciences, " and if their "nurture doesn't cost
too much. "[11]

Lederberg's one qualification to the program of mass cloning
would be that some individuals continue to be permitted to repro -
duce in the traditional way. There is a need that useful or
adaptive mutation continue to appear in the human race to suit
the changing environment. As they appear, they too can be
cloned to replace outmoded human models.

An Ethics for Genetic Manipulation

The revolutionary programs of eugenics or euphenics could
draw on Joseph Fletcher's modern "situation ethics" for philosophic underpinning. He holds with Jeremy Bentham that no
act, strictly speaking, can be evil in itself. He would decide
in every instance whether eugenic selection or cloning might
be good, and often enough he would decide yes:

> If the greatest good of the greatest number (i.e., the social
> good) were served by it, it would be justifiable not only to
> specialize the capacities of people by cloning or by constructive
> genetic engineering, but also to bio-engineer or bio-design
> parahumans or "modified men"--as chimeras (part animal) or
> cyborg-androids (part prostheses). I would vote for cloning
> top-grade soldiers and scientists, or for supplying them through
> other genetic means, if they were needed to offset an elitist or
> tyrannical power plot by other cloners--a truly science-fiction
> situation, but imaginable. I suspect I would favor making and
> using man-machine hybrids rather than genetically designed
> people for dull, unrewarding or dangerous roles needed none-
> theless for the community's welfare--perhaps the testing of sus-

pected pollution areas or the investigation of threatening vol-
canos or snow-slides.[12]

The guiding principles of a situation ethic, he says, are
teleological (goal oriented) rather than a priori (predetermined);
it is what works best for the most people. To be moral, scientific decisions need only be "tailored to a loving concern for
human beings. "[13] Yet there is evidence of an a priori principle
in his thinking. The same principle he considers is motivating
most scientific research: to be human is to make things work
better and, in the process, to master more of man's destiny.

> We cannot accept the "invisible hand" of blind natural chance
> or random nature in genetics any more that we could old Pro-
> fessor Javon's theory of feast and famine in 19th-century lais-
> sez faire economics, based on sun spots and tidal movements.
> To be men we must be in control. That is the first and last
> ethical word. For when there is no choice there is no pos-
> sibility of ethical action. Whatever we are compelled to do is
> amoral.[14]

By this line of reasoning he comes to the conclusion that scientifically manipulated reproduction is _more_ natural than the
traditional kind:

> It seems to me that laboratory reproduction is radically
> human compared to conception by ordinary heterosexual inter-
> course. It is willed, chosen, purposed and controlled, and
> surely these are among the traits that distinguished Homo
> sapiens from others in the animal genus, from the primates
> down. Coital reproduction is, therefore, less human than
> laboratory reproduction--more fun, to be sure, but with our
> separation of baby making from lovemaking, both become more
> human because they are matters of choice, and not chance.
> This is, of course, essentially the case for planned parenthood.
> I cannot see how either humanity or morality are served by
> genetic roulette.[15]

Moral Problems with Modern Eugenics

However lovingly the decision is made to clone a human being or engineer a biological hybrid, it nonetheless remains a
calculated decision by one person affecting another person's

biology. William T. Vukowich makes an exhaustive and sympathetic study of what seem to him to be the pressing social needs
that eugenics could serve very well, but comes somewhat re-
luctantly to the conclusion that authorities would have to impose
what might seem unconscionable controls to get it to work:

> Any... eugenics program is inherently discriminatory and
> thus raises a further constitutional issue. This inherent dis-
> crimination is invidious, based neither on what a person has
> done nor on anything over which he has control. The discrimi-
> nation in a eugenics program is based solely on a person's
> genetic heritage. Men might be born equal for some purposes,
> but they are not born genetically equal. A... eugenics program
> would require recognition of biological inequalities and abridge
> the fundamental rights of those declared genetically inferior.
> In this respect, eugenic legislation would parallel legislation
> of days gone by which imposed burdens on persons or denied
> them benefits because of their race. Both of these types of
> legislation impute intrinsic inferiority.[16]

Vukowich then goes on to say that such an imputation seems
to him nevertheless justified. He essentially adopts Fletcher's
line of reasoning that the common good justified abridging certain rights, among them the right to risk producing genetically
unsound children:

> But eugenics legislation would differ from racial legislation in
> a very important respect: legislation which denied benefits and
> imposed burdens on the basis of race was irrational because
> race is unrelated to a person's ability to perform, his merit,
> his contributions to society, or any other quality which would
> justify the discrimination. Eugenics legislation, however,
> would be rational: fundamental rights of persons would be
> abridged only to prevent their passing deleterious inheritable
> qualities to future generations....
>
> Although eugenics legislation would abridge fundamental
> civil rights and discriminate between persons on the basis of
> intrinsic characteristics, these factors alone should not render
> the legislation unconstitutional. Eugenics legislation, like other
> legislation which infringes on fundamental rights, would improve
> the quality of human life and help eliminate human suffering.[17]

(In the passage quoted Vukowich is speaking specifically about negative eugenics, but his remarks are appropriate about any program of eugenics; good breeding encouraged (positive eugenics) is bad breeding discouraged (negative eugenics). Both require coercion if in differing degrees. Muller's optimism about voluntary eugenics is not infectious.

The possible loss of free choice in breeding disquiets other writers more. Harold Green worries about the fearsome momentum of scientific research in this regard. He doesn't trust any current lack of scientific expertise or current legislative restrictions as assurance that artificial reproduction would not soon be with us, and then, thrust upon us. Science, he says, goes on doing its work inexorably, discovering systematically how to do whatever its visionary minds foresee. If the government supports the work (as the United States government often does), it becomes almost imperative that what is discovered be used. New laws follow hard upon breakthroughs.

> In the very nature of the political and bureaucratic processes, it is obvious that government officials will be reluctant to be cast in the position of having spent millions of dollars on research which serves no useful purpose. Thus, where the National Institutes of Health provide substantial funding for a particular area of research relating to "health," there are powerful pressures to see that the results are in fact used for "health." Similar interests and pressures exist with respect to the congressional sponsors of such research funding. When a resulting technology is ripe for application, the governmental sponsors adopt a classic form of advocacy: (1) use of the technology involves obvious and substantial benefits to the public health; (2) although there may be adverse consequences, we do not know this with certainty except in the light of experience with its use; (3) if experience demonstrates that there are adverse consequences, we may be able to eliminate or ameliorate the adverse effects through some other technological "fix"; (4) if the adverse consequences remain, we can enact regulatory laws which will enable us to benefit from the technology while appropriately minimizing the adverse effects; and (5) if all else fails, we can, of course, stop the use of the technology. It would appear to be axiomatic, therefore, that government sponsorship of a technology increases the inevitability that it will, in fact, be used, since the government's vested interest causes it to act more as promoter than resister.[18]

The most that Green can hope for is that the scientists involved in this kind of research might be willing to publicize
widely what they are up to. An educated public might be able
to at best "retard" progress to the point that they could absorb
its impact more gracefully.[19]   Interestingly, it is just this sort
of exposure that Lederberg fears for its unpredictable response:
"The precedents affecting the long-term rationale of social policy will be set not on the basis of well-debated principles, but
on the accident of the first advertised examples. The accidents
might be as capricious as the nationality, the batting average,
or public esteem of a clonant; the handsomeness of a parahuman
progeny; the private morality of the experimenters; or the public awareness that man is a part of the continuum of life."[20]

Paul Ramsey makes a more exclusively anthropological
criticism of eugenics, cloning, and in vitro fertilization. They
divorce the act of procreation from the act of love and thus would
wound humanity irrevocably: "The genetic proposal to clone a
man and the minority practice of artificial insemination from a
nonhusband donor are borderlines that throw into bold relief the
nature of human parenthood which both place under assault."[21]
He argues that human parenthood forms the last line of defense
of human nature. These techniques would tend to make the
purpose of marriage the breeding of superior stock; each technique would run the risk of producing experimental "mistakes"
that would have had no opportunity to consent or dissent from a
radical experiment on their body and lives; and even if a healthy
body were produced, who could predict the special loneliness
and alienation the first "artificial" persons would feel, cut off
from the traditional intimate bonds with living parents?

Ramsey explicitly criticizes Muller's argument that because
mankind is doomed unless positive steps are taken to regulate
our genetic endowment, such steps should be taken. He responds,
"The Christian knows no absolutely imperative end that would
justify any means...he will always have in mind the premise
that there may be a number of things that might succeed better
but would be intrinsically wrong means for him to adopt."[22] He
would have mankind die a natural death rather than kill its essential nature in trying to wrest off its genetic load. He responds
to Lederberg by repeating Lederberg's own reservations about
cloning--it rigidifies adaptability, increases the chances of

sterility, and runs the danger of making monstrosities if the
donor tissue cell is in a prolonged interphase condition while
the egg cell into which it is inserted is undergoing cleavage.
Ramsey adds that he finds the threat of creating monstrosities
to be cause not for caution but for prohibition of the whole process.

The whole range of genetic controls raises four questions
for Ramsey. The first is whether or not man has the wisdom
to be his own creator. Ramsey is pessimistic. "From man's
rape of the earth and his folly in exercising stewardship over
his environment by divine commission, there can be derived no
reason to believe that he ought now to reach for dominion over
the modifications of his own species. "[23] The second question asks
what the nature of human parenthood is and what the consequences
of its destruction would be. He responds that parenthood grounds
human nature in the flesh. Genetic control threatens to dominate
the flesh by reintroducing the outmoded ideas that mind and matter live apart: "The religious and moral traditions of the West
cannot subscribe to the sweeping notion that thought is superior
to the reality of the flesh, a notion manifest in most of these
dualistic 'mind in dominion over body' proposals. "[24] The third
question is whether humans should presume to play God. In so
doing Ramsey says they cease to play as humans, whose nature
it is to live with the world and body which circumstances not altogether unrandomly create: "... Man and his future may be at
stake when scientific messianists can now calmly contemplate
the utter removal or suppression of the human subject for the
sake of their own version of some future state of affairs--a future state they propose to create ex nihilo, or out of biological
components that do not take living men into respectful account. "[25]
The final question is whether man wouldn't be committing suicide
as a species if he persists in radically altering himself. An utterly
engineered human being is no more human than an insect or a god:
"... It is evident that, in the end and far, far earlier in the con-
verging lines of action leading to man's radical self-modification
and control of his evolutionary future, many of the proposals must
simply be described as a project for the suicide of the species.
The momentum behind them is despair over man as he is. "[26]

The only research into genetic engineering Ramsey would encourage would be genetic surgery. It offers to treat an afflicted
individual child for a particular malady. Its risks are the tra-

ditional ones of experimental medicine that can be and only should
be undertaken when they promise relief in extremis. It would
doctor an individual patient not as the other techniques would,
"that nonpatient, the human race."

Marc Lappé doesn't share Ramsey's absolute view that the
risk to the child should preclude in vitro fertilization. He sympa-
thizes with the parents. Once childless couples have been ap-
prised of all the foreseeable hazards of the procedure, he thinks
that they can assume responsibility for the risks to the fetus:

> If, in dissuading this kind of childbearing, one raises the spec-
> ter of "hidden dangers" and "unforeseeable consequences," he
> is using a specious moral argument. While it is imperative to
> weigh the extent and degree of foreseeable damage in vitro
> manipulations may produce, I recognize that we will only be
> able to pass judgment on the likely risks. Nevertheless, such
> an estimation can and must be made. What is necessary is to
> bring the evidence to bear on possible damage, to assess the
> risks and then to determine if at some point they fall to an
> acceptable level. In the case of human babies produced by in
> vitro procedures, presumably this level would be one which
> was equivalent to the risks normally undertaken in a "natural"
> pregnancy.[27]

Frank P. Grad suggests that perhaps new techniques of reproduction would bring them a perfectly legitimate if revolutionary concept of the family--a new moral context to justify it. The family would no longer be "a biologic unit composed
of a fertile male, a fertile female and children who are genetically theirs," but a "consensual unit wherein a man and a woman
who are married to each other agree to have and raise children,
to regard themselves and the children as family, and to give
each other the comfort of material and emotional support."[28]

John Batt, on the other hand, is as deeply suspicious as
Ramsey of any scientific meddling with the genetic process or
family life. He suspects that the scientists who do meddle
suffer from ill psychic health. "The well chronicled dedication of the epic heroes of science is, in the main, support for
my thesis that a virtue is quite often but the function of a
characterological necessity. It is likewise with the quest for

'superior being.' The urge to manufacture the genius Over-
man has its sources in unconscious feelings of ineffectuality
and the negative evaluation of self. Specifically, it derives
from one's failure to construct an adequate body image."[29] He
proposes healthy eroticism as the best defense against the unhealthy encroachments on human genetic integrity.

> The gambit of the privacy zone established by federal
> legislation must at a minimum circumscribe those aspects of
> being which promote personal expression; those aspects of
> being which allow a man to be free from the prescriptions of
> those who wish to convert him into a true believer. The triad
> of family, sexuality, and psyche form the best defense against
> authoritarianism. It is by guaranteeing the integrity of the
> family, one's freedom to determine one's own sexual exist-
> ence, and the right to form and explore one's inner space that
> we can preserve man's freedom and his ability to resist grand
> and petty tyranny.[30]

We close listening to a serene voice. Although the German
theologian Karl Rahner, like Ramsey and Batt, believes humans
would best remain mortal, fated, and tied to their growing and
aging flesh, unlike them he views the prospects of genetic engineering calmly. He acknowledges that these techniques threaten
humans with collective suicide. But he thinks such a thing isn't
likely to occur because "there is a framework which man has
not fashioned and which can never be transcended, or else it
would eliminate man as a historical being."[31] God is the framer;
whatever of autocreation humans can achieve, God would have
to co-sponsor. Therefore humans should proceed with confi-
dence, making whatever sacrifices are now needed for the sake
of the future generations. "Thus human autocreation will develop that concrete form of human openness which leads to the
absolute future that comes from God."[32] From this lofty perspective, it seems Rahner would look on the plans of scientists
such as Muller and Lederberg and say, "...There is really
nothing possible for man that he ought not do."[33]

Notes

Introduction

1.   See David H. Smith, "Theological Reflection and the New Biology, " <u>Indiana Law Journal</u> 48 (Summer 1973): 613, 615; and James M. Gustafson, "Genetic Engineering and the Normative View of the Human, " in <u>Ethical Issues in Biology and Medicine</u>, ed. Preston N. Williams (Cambridge, Mass.: Schenkman, 1973), pp. 48, 49.
2.   See Smith, pp. 615-16, n. 24, n. 26.
3.   <u>The New Yorker</u>, 6 March 1971.

Chapter One: Experimentation on Human Subjects

1.   See Leo Alexander, "Medical Science Under Dictatorship, " <u>The New England Journal of Medicine</u> 241 (14 July 1949): 39-47.
2.   See Elinor Langer, "Human Experimentation: Cancer Studies at Sloan-Kettering Stir Public Debate on Medical Ethics, " <u>Science</u> 143 (1964): 551 ff.
3.   For a discussion of these cases, see Richard M. Restak, <u>Pre-meditated Man: Bioethics and the Control of Human Life</u> (New York: Viking Press, 1975), pp. 111-23.
4.   See Barbara J. Culliton, "Fetal Research: The Case History of a Massachusetts Law, " <u>Science</u> 187 (24 January 1975): 237-41.
5.   Howard Hyatt, remarks made in the session "Future Policy Options and Summary, " <u>Experiments and Research with Humans</u>: Values in Conflict (Washington, D. C.: National Academy of Sciences, 1975), p. 217.
6.   David D. Rutstein, "The Ethical Design of Human Experiments, " <u>Daedalus</u> 98 (Spring 1969): 525.
7.   Guido Galabresi, "Reflections on Medical Experimentation in Humans, " <u>Daedalus</u> 98 (Spring 1969): 395.
8.   For reviews of the history of non-therapeutic research see Francis D. Moore, "Therapeutic Innovation: Ethical Boundaries in the Initial Clinical Trials of New Drugs and Surgical Procedures, " <u>Daedalus</u> 98 (Spring 1969): 502-22; and Francis D. Moore, "Perspectives of Biomedical Research: A Cultural and Historical View, " <u>Experiments and Research with Humans</u>, pp. 15-31.
9.   Paul Ramsey, <u>The Patient as Person: Explorations in Medical Ethics</u>

(New Haven: Yale University Press, 1970), pp. 5-6, 9.

10.   Margaret Mead, "Research with Human Beings: A Model Derived from Anthropological Field Practice," Daedalus 98 (Spring 1969): 374.

11.   Edmond Cahn, "The Lawyer as Scientist and Scoundrel: Reflections on Francis Bacon's Quadricentennial," New York University Law Review 36 (January 1961): 11.

12.   Hans Jonas, "Philosophical Reflections on Experimenting with Human Subjects," Daedalus 98 (Spring 1969): 226.

13.   Ibid, pp. 230, 231.

14.   Ibid, p. 237.

15.   Ibid.

16.   Ramsey, Patient as Person, p. 25.

17.   Alvin Bronstein, remarks in a session entitled "The Military/The Prisoner" at the conference of the National Academy of Science on Experiments and Research with Humans, published in Experiments and Research with Humans, p. 131.

18.   Galabresi, "Reflections," pp. 404-5.

19.   William J. Curran and Henry K. Beecher, "Experimentation in Children," The Journal of the American Medical Association 10 (6 October 1969): 83.

20.   See Louis Lasagna, "Special Subjects in Human Experimentation," Daedalus 98 (Spring 1969): 449-62, especially pp. 458, ff.

21.   Pp. 47, ff.

22.   Lasagna, "Special Subjects," p. 460.

23.   See Geoffrey Edsall, "A Positive Approach to the Problem of Human Experimentation," Daedalus 98 (Spring 1969): 463-79.

24.   Joseph Fletcher, "Pragmatists and Doctrinaires," The Hastings Center Report 5 (June 1975): 36-37.

25.   Ibid., p. 37.

26.   Gary L. Rebach, "Fetal Experimentation: Moral, Legal, and Medical Implications," Stanford Law Review 26 (May 1974): 1202.

27.   Leroy Walters, "Fetal Research and the Ethical Issues," The Hastings Center Report 5 (June 1975): 13-18.

28.   Richard Wasserstrom, "The Status of the Fetus," The Hastings Center Report 5 (June 1975): 19.

29.   Paul Ramsey, The Ethics of Fetal Research (New Haven: Yale University Press, 1975) p. 43.

30.   The Federal Register, vol. 40, no. 154 (8 August 1975): 33526-550. Some parts of the report had been published previously in The Hastings Center Report 5 (June 1975).

31.   Ibid., p. 33546.

32.   Ibid., p. 33549.

33.   Ramsey, Fetal Research, p. 40.

Chapter Two: Genetic Counseling and Screening

1.   F. Clarke Fraser, "Survey of Counseling Practices," in Ethical Issues in Human Genetics, ed. Bruce Hilton et al. (New York-London: Plenum Press, 1973), pp. 7-13.

2.   John Fletcher, "Parents in Genetic Counseling: The Moral Shape of Decision Making, " in Hilton et al. , p. 301.

3.   Ibid. , p. 311.

4.   Fraser, "Counseling Practices, " pp. 8-9, 11.

5.   Arno G. Motulsky, "Genetic Therapy: A Clinical Geneticists Response, "
in The New Genetics and the Future of Man, ed. Michael D. Hamilton (Grand
Rapids, Michigan: Eerdmans, 1973), p. 131.

6.   Paul Ramsey, "Screening: An Ethicist's View, "in Hilton et al. , p. 150.

7.   For a discussion of these last two cases see Richard M. Restak, Premeditated Man: Bioethics and the Control of Future Human Life, (New York:
Viking Press, 1975), pp. 80-84.

8.   From the case Salgo v. Leland Stanford, Jr. , University Board of Trustees,
cited in Philip R. Reilly, "Genetic Counselors and the Law, " Houston Law Review
12 (March 1975): 649.

9.   Alexander M. Capron, "Informed Decision Making in Genetic Counseling:
A Dissent to the 'Wrongful Life' Debate, " Indiana Law Journal 48 (Summer
1973): 592.

10.   H. J. Muller, "The Guidance of Human Evolution, " Perspectives in Biology
and Medicine, vol. 1 (Chicago: University of Chicago Press, 1959), p. 3.

11.   Fraser, "Counseling Practices, " p. 11.

12.   James Crow, "Population Perspective, " in Hilton et al. , p. 74. This article
gives a detailed analysis of the effects of genetic counseling on future generations.

13.   Robert S. Morison, "Implications of Prenatal Diagnosis for the Quality of,
and Right to, Human Life, " in Hilton et al. , p. 208.

14.   Fletcher, "Parents, " p. 326.

15.   Daniel Callahan, "The Meaning and Significance of Genetic Disease: Philosophical Perspectives, " in Hilton et al. , p. 89.

16.   Leon R. Kass, "Implications of Pre-natal Diagnosis for the Human Right
to Life, " in Hilton et al. , p. 193.

17.   Ibid. , p. 194.

18.   Ibid. , p. 196.

19.   Ibid. , p. 197.

20.   Ibid. , p. 198.

21.   See Frederick Ausubel, Jon Beckwith, and Kaaren Janseen, "The Politics
of Genetic Engineering: Who Decides Who's Defective?" Psychology Today
(June 1974).

22.   Marc Lappé and Richard Roblin, "Newborn Genetic Screening as a Concept
in Health Care Delivery, " Ethical, Social and Legal Dimensions of Screening
for Human Genetic Disease, vol. 10, no. 6 (1974), p. 4.

23.   Marc Lappé, "Moral Obligations and the Fallacies of 'Genetic Control,'"
Theological Studies 33 (September 1972): 411-27.

24.   Ramsey, "Screening, " p. 151.

25.   The New England Journal of Medicine 287 (1972): 204-5.

26.   John A. Osmundsen, "We Are All Mutants--Preventive Genetic Medicine: A
Growing Clinical Field Troubled by a Confusion of Ethicists, " Medical Dimensions
(February 1973), pp. 26-27.

27.   Ibid. , p. 28.

28.   Pages cited refer to the text of the report as contained in Amitai Etzioni, Genetic Fix (New York: Macmillan Co., 1973), pp. 240-49; first published in The New England Journal of Medicine 286 (25 May 1972): 1129-32.

29.   D. L. Stevens, "Tests for Huntington's Chorea,"New England Journal of Medicine 285, (1971): 413-14.

30.   Willard Gaylin, "Genetic Screening: The Ethics of Knowing," The New England Journal of Medicine 286 (1972): 1362.

Chapter Three: Abortion

1.   Daniel Callahan, Abortion: Law, Choice and Morality (London and New York: Macmillan, 1970), p. 290.

2.   Ibid., p. 292.

3.   Daniel Callahan, "Abortion: Some Ethical Issues, " in Abortion, Society and the Law, ed. David F. Walbert and J. Douglas Butler (Cleveland and London: The Press of Case Western Reserve University, 1973), p. 100.

4.   Ibid.

5.   Ibid., p. 99.

6.   Robert F. Drinan, S. J., "The Inviolability of the Right to be Born, " in Walbert and Butler, p. 132.

7.   Ibid., p. 130.

8.   Richard A. Schwartz, M.D., "Abortion on Request: the Psychiatric Implications, " in Walbert and Butler, p. 145.

9.   Ibid., p. 157.

10.   Ibid., pp. 164, 165, 166, 168.

11.   "Decisions of the United States Supreme Court in January 1973 with Respect to the Texas and Georgia Abortion Statutes, " in Walbert and Butler, p. 346.

12.   Ibid., p. 348.

13.   Ibid., p. 340-1.

14.   Ibid., p. 324.

15.   Ibid., p. 331.

16.   Richard McCormick, S.J., "Notes on Moral Theology: The Abortion Dossier, " Theological Studies (1973), p. 312.

17.   Judith Jarvis Thomson, "A Defense of Abortion, " Philosophy and Public Policy 1 (Fall 1971): 56,64.

18.   Sissela Bok, "Ethical Problems of Abortion, " Hastings Center Studies 2 (January 1974): 42.

19.   Ibid., p. 44.

20.   Baruch Brody, "Thomson on Abortion, " Philosophy and Public Affairs 2 (Spring 1972): 335-40.

21.   John Finnis, "The Rights and Wrongs of Abortion: A Reply to Judith Thomson, " Philosophy and Public Affairs 2 (Winter 1973): 123.

Chapter Four: Behavior Control — Psychotropic Drugs, Behavior Modification, and Psychosurgery

1.   See L. Risenberg et al., "A Psychopharmacologic Experiment in a Training School for Delinquent Boys," American Journal of Orthopsychiatry 33 (March 1963): 431-47.

2.   See Gerald C. Klerman, "Psychotropic Drugs as Therapeutic Agents," Hastings Center Report 2 (January 1974): 81-93.

3.   Lloyd H. Cotter, M.D., "Operant Conditioning in a Vietnamese Mental Hospital," American Journal of Psychiatry 124 (1967): 63.

4.   See O. T. Lovaas et al., "Acquisition of Imitative Speech by Schizophrenic Children," Science 151 (1966): 705-7.

5.   Vernon H. Mark, M.D., and Frank R. Ervin, M.D., Violence and the Brain (New York: Harper and Row, 1970), p. 97.

6.   Quoted in Peter R. Breggin, "The Return of Lobotomy and Psychosurgery," Quality of Health Care: Human Experimentation, 1973, Hearings before the U.S. Senate, Subcommittee on Health of the Committee on Labor and Public Welfare, 93rd Cong., 1st Sess., S. 974, S. 878, and S.J. Res.71, 23 February and 6 March 1973, part 2, pp. 456, 458.

7.   Ibid.

8.   Robert Veatch, "Drugs and Competing Drug Ethics," Hastings Center Studies 2 (January 1974): 68-80.

9.   Ibid., p. 72.

10.   Ibid., p. 75

11.   Ibid.

12.   Ibid., p. 76.

13.   Ibid., p. 78

14.   Lester Grinspoon and Susan B. Singer, "Amphetamines in the Treatment of Hyperkinetic Children," Harvard Educational Review 43 (November 1973): p. 518.

15.   Ibid., p. 546.

16.   Seymour L. Halleck, "Legal and Ethical Aspects of Behavior Control," The American Journal of Psychiatry 131 (1974): 384.

17.   Thomas S. Szasz, M.D., Ideology and Insanity: Essays on the Psychiatric Dehumanization of Man (Garden City: Anchor Books, 1970), p. 23.

18.   Robert Neville, "Ethical and Philosophical Issues of Behavior Control," a paper presented at the 139th Annual Meeting of the American Association for the Advancement of Science, 27 December 1972, reprint 804, Readings (Hastings-on-Hudson, N.Y.: Institute of Society, Ethics and the Life Sciences, n.d.

19.   Ibid., p. 6.

20.   Halleck, "Legal and Ethical Aspects," pp. 382, 383.

21.   Ibid., p. 383.

22.   Vernon H. Mark, M.D., and Robert Neville, Ph.D., "Brain Surgery in Aggressive Epileptics: Social Ethical Implications," The Journal of the American Medical Association 226 (1973): 767.

23.   Ibid., p. 768.

24.   Ibid., p. 771.

25.   Breggin, "Return of Lobotomy," p. 474.

26.   José M. R. Delgado, "Hell and Heaven within the Brain: the Systems for Punishment and Reward, " Physical Control of the Mind (1969); reprinted in Man Controlled: Readings in the Psychology of Behavior Control, ed. Marvin Karlins and Lewis M. Andrews (New York: The Free Press, 1972), p. 65.

27.   (New York: Harper Colophon, 1969), pp. 19-20.

28.   Ibid., p. 216.

29.   See Delgado, "Hell and Heaven, " pp. 63-64, 55ff.

30.   José M. R. Delgado, "Physical Manipulation of the Brain: A Special Supplement, " The Hastings Center Report (May 1973), pp. 3, 11.

31.   Breggin, "Return of Lobotomy, " p. 474.

32.   The Hastings Center Report, (May 1973), p. 7.

33.   Grinspoon and Singer, "Amphetamines, " p. 549.

34.   B. F. Skinner, Beyond Freedom and Dignity, (New York: Bantam, 1972), p. 19.

35.   Ibid., pp. 153-54.

36.   Ibid., p. 157.

37.   John R. Platt, "The Skinnerian Revolution, " in Beyond the Punitive Society, ed. Harvey Wheeler, (San Francisco: W. H. Freeman and Company, 1973), p. 42.

38.   Romans 7: 19.

39.   Platt, "Skinnerian Revolution, " p. 48.

40.   Ibid., p. 50

41.   B. F. Skinner, Walden Two (New York: Macmillan, 1962), pp. 296, 297.

42.   Carl R. Rogers and B. F. Skinner, "Some Issues Concerning the Control of Human Behavior: A Symposium, " Science 124 (30 November 1956): 1057-66; reprinted in Marvin Karlins and Lewis M. Andrews, p. 253.

43.   Ibid., p. 257.

44.   Ibid., p. 258.

45.   Ibid., p. 261.

46.   Ibid., p. 263.

47.   Willard Gaylin, "Skinner Redux, " Harper's Magazine (October 1973), pp. 48-56.

48.   Ibid., p. 54.

49.   Neville, "Ethical and Philosophical Issues, " p. 10.

50.   Gerald Leach, The Biocrats: Implications of Medical Progress (Baltimore: Penguin Books, 1972), p. 233.

51.   Ibid., p. 204.

52.   Ibid., p. 210.

Chapter Five: Death and Dying —
New Criteria for Death, Heroic Medicine,
Organ Transplants, and Euthanasia

1.   Gerald Leach, The Biocrats: Implications of Medical Progress (Baltimore: Penguin, 1972), p. 312.

2.   "A Definition of Irreversible Coma, " Report of the Ad Hoc Committee of the Harvard Medical School to Examine the Definition of Brain Death, The Journal of the American Medical Association 205 (5 August 1968): 338.

3.   J. B. Brierly et al., "Neocortical Death after Cardiac Arrest, " The Lancet (11 September 1971), p. 565.

4.   Robert S. Morison, "Death: Process or Event?" Science 173 (20 August 1971): 696, 697.

5.   Leon R. Kass, "Death as an Event: A Commentary on Robert Morison, " Science 173 (20 August 1971): 698-702.

6.   Hans Jonas, Philosophical Essays: From Ancient Creed to Technological Man (Englewood Cliffs, N. J.: Prentice-Hall, 1974), pp. 138, 139.

7.   Ibid. , p. 139.

8.   David D. Rutstein, "The Ethical Design of Human Experimentation, " Daedalus 98 (Spring 1969): 5.

9.   "Refinements in Criteria for the Determination of Death: An Appraisal, " The Journal of the American Medical Association 221 (3 July 1972): 48-53.

10.   Ibid., p. 53.

11.   Ibid., p. 52.

12.   Walter S. Ross, "Clinical Research Is the Best Medicine, " Medical Opinion (February 1972), p. 52, 55.

13.   Quoted in Time, 3 November 1961, p. 60; discussed in Paul Ramsey, The Patient as Person: Explorations in Medical Ethics (New Haven: Yale University Press, 1970), pp. 146-48.

14.   Herman Feifel et al., "Physicians Consider Death, " Proceedings, 75th Annual Convention, American Psychological Association, (1967), pp. 201-2.

15.   Ibid., p. 202.

16.   Donald Oken, M.D., "What to Tell Cancer Patients, " The Journal of the American Medical Association 175 (1 April 1961): 1126.

17.   Ivan Illich, "The Political Uses of Natural Death, " Hastings Center Studies 2 (January 1974): 3.

18.   William F. May, "The Sacral Power of Death in Contemporary Experience, " Social Research 39 (Autumn 1972): 488.

19.   Ramsey, Patient as Person, p. 126.

20.   Ibid.

21.   Ibid., pp. 161, 162.

22.   Hon. Michael T. Sullivan, "The Dying Person -- His Plight and His Right, " New England Law Review 8 (Spring 1973): 197-216; see notes on p. 210 ff.

23.   Ibid., p. 216.

24.   George Fletcher, "Prolonging Life, " Washington Law Review 42 (1967): 1015.

25.   Cited in ibid., p. 1014.

26.   Cited in The Hastings Center Report 6 (February 1976): 8.

27.   Thomas C. Oden, "Beyond an Ethic of Immediate Sympathy, " ibid., p. 13.

28.   Melvin D. Levine, "Disconnection: The Clinician's View, " ibid., p. 12.

29.   Alexander Capron, "Shifting the Burden of Decision-Making, " ibid., p. 19.

30.   "In the Matter of Karen Quinlan, An Alleged Incompetent, " argued 26 January 1976, decided 31 March 1976, in New Jersey Superior Court, Chancery Division, reported at 137 N. J. Super. 227 (1976).

31.   Ibid., p. 49.

32. Ibid., pp. 57-58.

33. Elizabeth Kübler-Ross, On Death and Dying (New York: Macmillan Co., 1973), pp. 9-10.

34. Ibid., p. 276.

35. "Definition of Irreversible Coma." p. 339.

36. Kass, "Death as Event," p. 701.

37. Jesse Dukeminier and David Sanders, "Organ Transplantation: A Proposal for Routine Salvaging of Cadaver Organs," New England Journal of Medicine 79 (1968): 413-19.

38. News about Uniform Anatomical Gift Act (New York: Natural Transplant Information Center, United Health Foundations, 1969).

39. Ramsey, Patient as Person, p. 210.

40. William May, "Attitudes Toward the Newly Dead," Hastings Center Studies 1, no. 1 (1973) : 6.

41. Leach, Biocrats, p. 315.

Chapter Six: Allocation of Scarce Medical Resources

1. Edmond Cahn, The Moral Decision: Right and Wrong in the Light of American Law (Bloomington: Indiana University Press, 1955), p. 71.

2. Leo Shatin, "Medical Care and the Social Worth of a Man," American Journal of Orthopsychiatry 36 (1967): 100.

3. Shana Alexander, "They Decide Who Lives, Who Dies," Life 53 (9 November 1962): 102-28.

4. David Sanders and Jesse Dukeminier, Jr., "Medical Advance and Legal Lag: Hemodialysis and Kidney Transplantation," UCLA Law Review 15 (February 1968): 364.

5. Paul A. Freund, "Introduction to the Issue 'Ethical Aspects of Experimentation with Human Subjects,'" Daedalus 98 (Spring 1969): xiii.

6. Paul Ramsey, The Patient as Person: Explorations in Medical Ethics (New Haven: Yale University Press, 1970), p. 247.

7. Ibid., pp. 265-66.

8. See Paul Freund in Daedalus and also Henry K. Beecher, "Scarce Resources and Medical Advancement," Daedalus 98 (Spring 1969): 280.

9. James F. Childress, "Who Shall Live When Not All Can Live," Soundings 43 (Winter 1970): 335-39.

10. Frederic B. Westervelt, Jr., M.D., "A Reply to Childress: The Selection Process as Viewed from Within," Soundings 43 (Winter 1970): 362.

11. Ramsey, Patient as Person, p. 268.

12. Gerald Leach, The Biocrats (Baltimore: Penguin, 1970) p. 353.

13. Beecher, "Scarce Resources," p. 307.

14. Ramsey, Patient as Person, p. 274.

15. Leach, Biocrats, p. 344.

16. Ibid., p. 330.

17. Paul Starr, "The Politics of Therapeutic Nihilism," The Hastings Center Report 6 (October 1976): 28.

18. Evelyn M. Kitagawa and Philip M. Hauser, Differential Mortality: A Study in Socioeconomic Epidemiology (Cambridge: Harvard University Press, 1973), p. 11; cited in Starr, "Therapeutic Nihilism," p. 27.

19. Ivan Illich, Medical Nemesis: The Expropriation of Health (New York: Pantheon, 1976); cited in Starr, "Therapeutic Nihilism," p. 25.

20. Starr, "Therapeutic Nihilism," p. 29.

21. (Cambridge: M.I.T. Press, 1974).

22. Rutstein, Blueprint, p. 174.

23. Paul Starr, "A National Health Program: Organizing Diversity," The Hastings Center Report 1 (February 1975): 12.

24. Ibid., p. 13.

Chapter Seven: The Eugenic Medicine of the Future Through In Vitro Fertilization, Genetic Surgery, and Cloning

1. For a discussion of the industrial possibilities of the new biology, see James F. Danielli, "Industry, Society and Genetic Engineering," The Hastings Center Report 2 (December 1972): 507, ff.

2. Willard Gaylin, "Genetic Screening: The Ethics of Knowing," New England Journal of Medicine 286 (1972): 1361.

3. For a discussion of the difficulties of coercing a mass application of new biological techniques, see Bernard D. Davis, "Prospects for Genetic Intervention in Man," Science 170 (1970): 1279-83, esp. pp. 1281-82.

4. Nicholas Wade, "Genetics: Conference Sets Strict Controls to Replace Moratorium," Science 187 (14 March 1975): 931.

5. See Lorence L. Bravenec, "Law and the Modification of Heredity Through DNA Chemistry," Journal of Family Law 8 (1968): 13-40.

6. H. J. Muller, "The Guidance of Human Evolution," in Perspectives in Biology and Medicine, vol. 1 (Chicago: University of Chicago Press, 1959) p. 3.

7. H. J. Muller, "Our Load of Mutations," The American Journal of Human Genetics 2 (June 1950): 146.

8. H. J. Muller, "The Guidance of Human Evolution," in Perspectives, vol. 3, p. 37.

9. Joshua Lederberg, "Experimental Genetics and Human Evolution," Bulletin of the Atomic Scientists 22 (October 1966): 5, 6.

10. Ibid., p. 9.

11. Ibid., p. 11.

12. Joseph Fletcher, "Ethical Aspects of Genetic Controls," New England Journal of Medicine 285 (1971): 779.

13. Ibid., p. 789.

14. Ibid., p. 782.

15. Ibid., p. 781

16. William T. Vukowich, "The Dawning of the Brave New World--Legal, Ethical, and Social Issues of Eugenics," University of Illinois Law Forum (1971): 208.

17.   Ibid., p. 209.
18.   Harold P. Green, "Genetic Technology: Law and Policy for the Brave New World," Indiana Law Journal 48 (Summer 1973): 576.
19.   Ibid., p. 579.
20.   Lederberg, "Experimental Genetics," p. 11.
21.   Paul Ramsey, Fabricated Man: The Ethics of Genetic Control (New Haven and London: Yale University Press, 1970), pp. 86-87.
22.   Ibid., p. 30.
23.   Ibid., p. 124.
24.   Ibid., p. 135.
25.   Ibid., p. 142
26.   Ibid., p. 159.
27.   Marc Lappé, "Risk-taking for the Unborn," The Hastings Center Report 2 (February 1972): 2.
28.   Frank P. Grad, "Legislative Responses to the New Biology: Limits and Possibilities," UCLA Law Review 15 (Fall 1968): 494.
29.   John Batt, "They Shoot Horses, Don't They: An Essay on the Scotoma of One-Eyed Kings," UCLA Law Review 15 (Fall 1968): 513.
30.   Ibid., p. 546.
31.   Karl Rahner, "Experiment: Man," Science and Faith in the 21st Century, ed, Donald Brophy (New York: Paulist Press, 1968), p. 37.
32.   Ibid., p. 33.
33.   Ibid., p. 22.

Index